MEDICINE

UNBUNDLED

MEDICINE UNBUNDLED

A JOURNEY THROUGH THE MINEFIELDS
OF INDIGENOUS HEALTH CARE

Gary Geddes

VICTORIA · VANCOUVER · CALGARY

Heritage House Publishing Company Ltd.
heritagehouse.ca

CATALOGUING INFORMATION AVAILABLE FROM LIBRARY AND ARCHIVES CANADA

978-1-77203-164-5 (pbk)
978-1-77203-165-2 (epub)
978-1-77203-166-9 (epdf)

Edited by Lara Kordic
Proofread by Lenore Hietkamp
Cover and interior book design by Jacqui Thomas
Cover photos courtesy of Joan Morris

The interior of this book was produced on 100% post-consumer recycled paper, processed chlorine free, and printed with vegetable-based inks.

We acknowledge the financial support of the Government of Canada through the Canada Book Fund (CBF) and the Canada Council for the Arts, and the Province of British Columbia through the British Columbia Arts Council and the Book Publishing Tax Credit.

Canadä BRITISH COLUMBIA BRITISH COLUMBIA ARTS COUNCIL
An agency of the Province of British Columbia

21 20 19 18 17   1 2 3 4 5

Printed in Canada

This book is dedicated to the Indigenous peoples of this land and to those newcomers with open hearts who will come to love them.

"If I am given this world with its injustices, it is not so that I might contemplate them coldly, but that I might animate them with my indignation." —JEAN-PAUL SARTRE

Table of Contents

PART THREE
The Long Sentence—And the First Shall Be Last

PART FOUR
Restoring the Song—Lessons for the Hard of Hearing

Acknowledgements

I 'd like to acknowledge the friendship, generosity, and help provided by so
many people over the four years this book has been taking shape. In the
case of Joan Morris, this involved numerous enjoyable, troubling, and instructive encounters, during which some of my ignorance of Indigenous history and
values was chipped away and a deep friendship and mutual respect developed.
Others, like Nancy Gibson, John Whittaker, Clifford Cardinal, Alice Ridout,
Ed Sadowski, James Daschuk, Linda McDonald, Marilyn Murray-Allison, Gary
Bosgoed, Yvonne Boyer, Kim Recalma-Clutesi, and Adam Dick went out of their
way to host, educate, and encourage me. I am grateful to them and others who
trusted me enough to share their ideas and experiences, through emails, phone
calls, and in person: Eleanor James-Robertson, Roger Ellis, Margaret Nachshen
(for the inspiration of and permission to reprint her etching), Lorraine Yuzicapi,
Rick Favel, Annie Smith St. Georges, André-Robert St. Georges, Saul Day,
Theodore Fontaine, Niigaanwewidam James Sinclair, Belvie Brebber, Melinda
Bullshields, Shirley Horn, Gloria Nicolson, Mike Cachagee, Noel Starblanket,
Richard McCutcheon, Chief Robert Joseph, Velvet Maud, Jennifer Mackie, Bill
Asikinack, Jonathan Dewar, Amy Bombay, Mary Nicholas, Alex McComber,
Albert McLeod, Krista McCracken, Jim Anderson, Stephen Carney, Jody Porter,
Albert Dumont, Graham Porter, David Haogak, Mervin Joe, Debbie Gordon
Ruben, Catherine Cockney, Gregory Brass, Beverly Amos, Tom O'Flanagan,
Irene Lindsay, Edward Chamberlain, Dale Burkholder, Margery Fee, Claudia
Malacrida, Daniel Josh Rowe, Peter Twohig, Wayne K. Spear, Carol Harrison,

9

Debbie Bookchin, Jim Schumacher, Monique Gray Smith, Miranda Jimmy, Keavy Martin, Lauren McKeon, Danielle Metcalfe-Chenail, George Muldoe, Rayanne Doucet, Karl Hele, Linc Kessler, Carl Urion, and Roy Little Chief. Several people, including Yvonne Boyer, Suzanne Fournier, Nancy Gibson, Rosalyn Boyd, my wife Ann Eriksson, Daniel Coleman, Warren Cariou, Paul DePasquale, and Alice Ridout generously read and commented on the manuscript, saving me from mistakes, misunderstandings, and more than a few graceless moments.

I am especially grateful to the many authors I read, some of whom are quoted extensively in this book. Among them, Suzanne Fournier, James Daschuk, and Maureen Lux deserve a special word of thanks. Suzanne Fournier's *Stolen from Our Embrace*, which she co-authored with Ernie Crey, was one of the first and most powerful books I read. James Daschuk's *Clearing the Plains* knocked my socks off with its passion and insights into the brutal and nefarious campaign to displace the Indigenous peoples of the prairies. And Maureen Lux's *Medicine That Walks* informed and inspired me throughout my research and writing. Her brilliant and detailed analysis of the motivations for and the history and legacy of Canada's segregated Indian hospitals, *Separate Beds*, was unfortunately not released until a week or two before my own research and writing had wound down. For anyone who wants to go deeper into the disturbing story of Indigenous health and wellbeing in Canada, I cannot recommend her new book too highly.

It's a tradition, which I'm glad to share, for writers to thank their long-suffering partners. Joseph Conrad's wife, Jesse, left his meals outside the door so as not to disturb the "genius" at his desk. My case is thankfully quite different: no genius, just hard work. My wife Ann Eriksson and I not only shared all the cooking and ate our meals together, but also inspired each other by knuckling down on our respective manuscripts. Her dedication in the research, writing and endless polishing of her fifth novel, *The Performance*, inspired and sometimes shamed me, for which I am truly grateful.

I want to thank, as well, the staff at Heritage House, including my editor, Lara Kordic, and my publisher, Rodger Touchie, who had faith in this project and offered me a contract after the larger presses in the country had said either "This is an important subject, Gary, but we'd never be able to sell it," or "Sadly, no one in Canada is interested in Indians."

Introduction _____

What prompts a paleface, and a wrinkled one at that, to write a book about Indigenous health issues in a climate where political correctness reigns and where such folly is likely to be dismissed on all sides as cultural appropriation or worse? I knew the risks of embarking on a project such as this before I began. I was even warned by a few friends and well-meaning specialists that I might end up looking like St. Sebastian, often depicted as a sad and saintly human pincushion shot through with arrows, or like someone who's tried to tango with a porcupine. I made similar questionable forays into sub-Saharan Africa in 2008 and 2009, hoping to learn something about justice and healing, how those suffering from the effects of poverty, genocide, and war managed to reconstruct at least the semblance of a normal life. While in northern Uganda, I interviewed an Acholi woman named Nancy, who had had her ears, nose, and lips cut off by the Lord's Resistance Army. As she spoke to me through an interpreter, I couldn't help comparing her story to the situation of Indigenous people back home, where many are living, and dying, in what some have called Fourth World conditions, their bodies dumped in rivers or left frozen outside cities by racist police, neglected children sniffing glue and committing suicide on over-crowded, polluted, postage-stamp reserves, all in one of the most privileged countries in the world.

An abbreviated answer to the question posed above might be this: outrage at what is still happening to Indigenous peoples in Canada, and at my own complicity, set me on this path. More importantly, I was invited to write this book by Joan Morris, an Indigenous acquaintance who, along with members of her family, was grievously mistreated at the Nanaimo Indian Hospital on Vancouver Island. My interviews with Joan led not only to a rich friendship, but also to more in-depth research on a subject about which I had known nothing. It's a long and intriguing story and one that, as the casualties mounted, took me to Yukon, the Northwest Territories, and across Canada several times between 2012 and 2016. But first, let me share a few thoughts about the so-called "Indian hospitals" and how history gets written.

Concern for Indigenous health is a relatively recent phenomenon in Canada. Subjugation or extermination seem to have been the only two options open to Indigenous peoples when the Spanish and other Europeans decided to occupy North and South America after 1492. Guns were the principal means of delivering this message, and superior technology has a way of making invaders consider themselves superior as well. So, if disease, accidentally or deliberately spread, carried off a large percentage of the original inhabitants, so much the better. The remainder would be useful as slaves, "country wives," guides, and manual labour. In Canada-to-be, to avoid conflict and possible defeat in some areas north of the 49th parallel, where the Indigenous populations outnumbered the settlers, treaties were signed that offered, or at least implied, respect, medical care, and assorted assistance in exchange for shared use of land. Although it seems obvious that many government signatories did not consider the offer of medical chests a serious long-term commitment to Indigenous health, the chiefs and their people certainly did. And when they started to die in epidemics of smallpox, flu, polio, and tuberculosis, and those promises were not kept, trust was all but destroyed.

But the vanishing people somehow survived, along with their medical afflictions, and certain groups—who had as much interest in souls as in bodies—began to attend to these ailments. From the time the Catholic Grey Nuns opened a hospital on the Blood Reserve in 1893 until the last government-run segregated Indian hospital was closed in 1996 at Fort Qu'Appelle, Saskatchewan, the separate system accounted for more than twenty Indian hospitals—especially if you include residential schools, such as St. Michael's in Alert Bay, that had medical facilities attached called preventoria. What they prevented was not the spread of disease but the loss of revenue from sick students being transferred elsewhere. In addition to three facilities in Ontario (Moose Factory Indian Hospital, Sioux Lookout Indian Hospital, and the Fort William Indian Hospital Sanatorium), the bulk of the segregated hospitals, fifteen to be exact, were in western Canada: five in Manitoba, one in Saskatchewan, six in Alberta, and five in British Columbia. Their heyday, from 1946 to 1967, as I was destined to learn, was not a great source of pride for the country.

Apprehension of sick Indigenous people was made legal by the Indian Act. Not yet having achieved the status of "persons," never mind citizens of Canada, they were susceptible to quarantine or incarceration at the whim of doctors, Indian agents, or government officials. Declaring individuals contagious was a good means of control, keeping them out of trouble or out of circulation while the task of clearing the land was underway.

My ambition in writing this book was to contact Elders from most of these institutions, but it quickly became clear that many of the survivors had already passed away and that displacement, starvation, humiliation, betrayal, residential schools, and what might be described—a gross under-statement, at best—as second-rate health care, had eroded the willingness of Indigenous peoples to talk to yet another non-Indigenous researcher, however sympathetic he may be. A hundred emails and phone calls to band councils did not open a single door. I learned the hard, and the slow, way that word-of-mouth contact is the only way of establishing the kind of trust that makes sharing stories possible. So I let friends, research, social contacts, and serendipity dictate my next move. As things progressed slowly, I was able to read widely, spend more time with certain individuals, and pay closer attention to what I found on the page and to what thirty-four Elders were saying by phone, in emails, and in person.

In the process, this project morphed from a narrow study of the seg-regated Indian hospitals to a broader consideration of the impediments—I have come view them as "minefields"—in the way of Indigenous health, including not only the negative list I've provided in the previous paragraph, but also the underlying and systemic racism that fuels them. The insights of Maureen Lux, James Daschuk, Mary-Ellen Kelm, Yvonne Boyer, and more than a dozen others who have written about Indigenous health have also helped to push me in this direction.

According to Italian writer and thinker Benedetto Croce, "Where there is no narrative, there is no history."[1] This comment has always intrigued me for its reminder that our lives are governed by the stories with which we surround ourselves, both personally and collectively. At the personal level, self-defining narratives are subject to constant change, corrected by new information and new needs, or distorted out of guilt, embarrassment, fear, or a failing memory. Details and emphases change, depending on whom we talk to.

With nations, it's a different process altogether. The national narrative has a tendency to become rigid, resistant to change or emendation. After 1867, Canada's national narrative was one of youth: "O Child of nations, giant-limbed," the poet sang.[2] Later, another misguided songbird would insist "it's only by our lack of ghosts we're haunted."[3] Along with ideas of youth and newness came the notion of innocence—as if, like Adam and Eve, we started with a clean slate in an empty land—which portrays Canadians as a "gentle people," a nation of peacekeepers, and our country as number one destination for the wretched of the earth. In this view, anything bad that happens to challenge the prevailing narrative is either ignored or dismissed as the work of a few bad apples.

Whether he believed it or not at the time, former prime minister Stephen Harper contributed to this myth of innocence. At a news conference in 2009, after the G20 Summit in Pittsburgh, he told his audience, "We also have no history of colonialism. So we have all of the things that many people admire about the great powers but none of the things that threaten or bother them."[4] Had he buried his head in the sand, like George Bush on the subject of Iraq, or was he just playing to foreign ignorance? A year earlier, he had made an official apology in Parliament to the Indigenous peoples of this land, not including those in Newfoundland and Labrador, for the travesty of government-funded, church-run residential schools. Is it possible he still believed there was no link between these racist institutions and their colonial origins, that these schools were simply the bad application of good policy?

14
—

A country's real history is not to be found in its dominant narrative or public pronouncements, but in the book of its deeds. Any serious historian of Canada can fill pages with atrocious deeds committed by the colonizers who appropriated this land and subsequent governments that ruled it. An abbreviated list might include the Head Tax inflicted on Chinese immigrants; the incarceration of Japanese-Canadians and theft of their property during World War II; continuous police and military actions against miners, strikers, environmental activists, minorities, and the poor; and the turning away in Vancouver of the *Komagata Maru* and its cargo of Sikhs in 1913 and a shipload of Jews in flight from the coming Holocaust on board the *St. Louis* in 1939, refused entry to Canada because politicians and bureaucrats in Ottawa thought one Jew was too many. More recently, we have added to this shameful list the torture and murder of Somali teenager Shidane Abukar Arone by members of the Canadian Airborne Regiment and the rendition and torture of Maher Arar. These were not random events perpetrated by a few bad apples, but the products of systemic racism.

Noticeably absent from the above list, and presumably from Harper's mind in 2009, are several centuries of travesties against the Indigenous peoples—not just the Beothuks, forced from their coastal food supply and hunted to extinction in Newfoundland, but also the great tribes who welcomed, fought alongside us, and shared their land only to be starved, betrayed, displaced, infected, and humiliated. Canada, if the national narrative were to include the real story, might be recognized globally as the world's largest and most successful land-grab, a nasty, brutish, ongoing piece of work. This land was not, when the settlers arrived, a *tabula rasa*, a blank slate ripe for inscription; it was an ancient land, inhabited throughout by self-sufficient, sophisticated peoples, with laws, customs, art, rituals, and their own history and myths of origin. There was no lack of ghosts, had we bothered to look for and acknowledge them. And some of these ghosts are now demanding to be heard.

As a result of our refusal to rewrite the national narrative, the exploitation of Canada's Indigenous peoples continues to result in broken lives, dysfunctional families, and devastated communities. It's true that we have our strengths, but we cannot mature as a nation if we insist on living a lie or a half-truth. We need to rewrite our history, accept responsibility, and

15

make sure it never happens again, which means acknowledging the dark or shadow-side of our past and present. Politicians and journalists, and each new generation, need to know the truth about our collective past, so no one is foolish enough to suggest that Canada lost its innocence at Ypres or Vimy Ridge, or when a lone gunman entered the House of Commons. As playwright and political scientist Herschel Hardin suggested in 1974 in *A Nation Unaware*: "Creating a simulacrum of innocence is only a way colonials have of avoiding their condition."[5]

The process of rewriting the national narrative to include the real history of our relations with the First Peoples of this land is already underway, thanks to the writings of many Indigenous and non-Indigenous authors, including Harold Cardinal, Suzanne Fournier, Ernie Crey, James Daschuk, Yvonne Boyer, Maureen Lux, Tom King, Laurie Meijer Drees, Marilyn Dumont, Joseph Boyden, Mary-Ellen Kelm, Tomson Highway, Louise (Sky Dancer) Halfe, Richard Wagamese, and many others. Unfortunately, too few Canadians have read their books and too few of the truths offered have made their way into our history texts. However, it's becoming more difficult to pretend we're innocents now that the chief justice of the Supreme Court of Canada, the Right Honourable Beverley McLachlin, and the Honourable Justice Murray Sinclair, head of the Truth and Reconciliation Commission (TRC), have joined the growing list of those using the word "genocide" to describe the Canada's long-standing treatment of First Nations, Inuit, and Métis.

What follows is a hard but hopeful look at the troubling state of health amongst Canada's Indigenous peoples and an examination of its causes. Not just the Indian Act, the residential schools and the segregated and under-funded Indian hospitals, but also the systemic racism that is still the principal driving force that allowed Brian Sinclair to die in an emergency ward in a Winnipeg hospital, after sitting alone and unattended in his wheelchair for thirty-four hours; that made it possible for Ivan Morris to be operated on and left for dead in the morgue of the Nanaimo Indian Hospital; that enabled Richard Thomas's killer at Kuper Island Residential School to go unpunished; that tolerated the use of children as sexual objects

16

and guinea pigs in residential schools and segregated hospitals; that turns a blind eye on the fact that more than twelve hundred Indigenous women and girls have gone missing or murdered for more than a decade without an official inquiry; and that, even now, overlooks countless others living in poverty, polluted environments, and over-crowded and decrepit housing.

When I think of doctors, the first, somewhat antiquated, image that comes to mind is the small black leather bag that contains a stethoscope, tongue depressors, gauze, bandages, splints, assorted pieces of equipment, and some basic medications. Indigenous medicine has its own images: the shaman or healer, widely versed in the healing properties of plants, and the traditional medicine bundle, which contains precious items of spiritual significance intended to foster protection, good luck, and healing: tobacco, bones, seeds, herbs, feathers, teeth, and other relics with a personal or tribal significance. When the bundles were confiscated and either destroyed or left to moulder in museums, their powers, including the power to fend off or mitigate suffering, were lost to the individual and the community. Medicine bundles remind me, in reverse, of Pandora's box which, when opened, released illness, misfortune, and death into the world. The medicine bundle, by contrast, contains healing energies—physical, mental, and spiritual—that we all, not only Indigenous people, desperately need. However, there is one thing the medicine bundle and Pandora's box have in common.

At the bottom of Pandora's box, as a possible antidote to the evils released into the world, is that most precious of human commodities: hope. The medicine bundle, in addition to its other healing properties, is, above all, a repository of hope. So, too, the sharing of personal experiences provides a way of releasing that hope and its healing powers. The stories unbundled and made available in this book are testaments to the courage and hope of segregated hospital and residential school survivors, generously shared so we can all begin to heal and learn to live together as equals, as brothers and sisters.

I want to thank Songhees Elder Joan Morris, who shared the first of many hospital experiences related in this book and who set me on this path, at times a steep learning curve, though she's not responsible for the moments of stumbling and misunderstanding that follow. *Medicine*

17

Unbundled, which would not exist without her, is as much her book as it is mine. Joan's survival, like that of many in her own and previous generations, is not only a miracle, but also a story of resilience. As difficult as it has been for me, and will be for you as a reader, to confront some of these testimonies, the integrity, humour, and grace under fire of the survivors who shared them is good reason for us all to hope.

PART ONE

JOANIE'S PEOPLE

Discarding the Masks
of Shame

one

Intertidal Zone

As waters ebb from the tidal flat in front of my house on Thetis Island, small boat traffic diminishes to nothing. Two major sandbars on either side of the central channel slowly break the surface, and beyond them several tiny serpentine estuaries begin to drain, leaving in the early morning sun drying shapes that resemble dunes. Bordered by second-growth forest, these sandbars are a far cry from the mental landscapes that have preoccupied me for the past four years, the jungles and semi-deserts of sub-Saharan Africa. Yet a few hundred yards beyond that tree line on neighbouring Penelakut Island (formerly known as Kuper) lie the remnants of a community shelled by British warships, ravaged by a residential school and systemic racism, and devastated by infectious diseases.

I've been trying to pull together some ideas for a lecture on Africa, but thoughts of the Kuper Island Residential School are making that impossible. Instead, I'm reading everything about Indigenous history I can lay my hands on, including Suzanne Fournier's and Ernie Crey's *Stolen from Our Embrace: The Abduction of First Nations Children and the Restoration of Aboriginal Communities*, a powerful indictment of the residential school system and an important source of ideas for the road ahead. The book is a seamless weaving of research, commentary, and interviews with survivors of the residential schools and the Sixties Scoop, the term now used to refer to the government policy of taking Indigenous children and farming them out to foster homes and for adoption by non-Indigenous families. The book not only details atrocities committed on Penelakut Island, an account so graphic and moving it is painful to read, but also comments on the origins and lethal objectives of the residential schools elsewhere in the province and throughout the country, institutions that BC Supreme Court Justice Douglas Hogarth rightly described as "institutionalized pedophilia."

Crey and Fournier address the legacy of residential schools on the physical and mental health of Indigenous peoples, especially the resultant intergenerational trauma and its devastating trajectory of sexual abuse, alcoholism, and suicide in so many families and communities. They explain the former as survivors' unconscious attempts to "take back their power by victimizing their loved ones as they had been victimized,"[1] and they quote Musqueam leader Wendy Grant-John, one-time contender for the position of AFN National Chief, who describes residential schools as "internment camps."[2] For all the suffering Fournier and Crey so painstakingly document, and for which they suggest positive approaches, what touches me most is their portrayal of the gradual re-emergence of the Indigenous courage, determination, and pride that has helped save countless lives and fuel so much inspiring grassroots activism.

I realize not only how ill-equipped I still am to be talking about complex and distant realities in Africa, but also how acutely unaware I am of what has been happening in my own backyard. So on April 13, 2012, I've arranged to spend the day with my daughter Bronwen at the Truth and Reconciliation Commission hearings in Victoria, where survivors of Canada's residential schools will be sharing the painful truths of their encounters with the colonial project now known as Canada. The hearings are being held—with what I will come to recognize as subtle Indigenous irony—in a conference centre attached to the famous Empress Hotel.

Bronwen has just joined the Department of Indian Affairs and is keen to learn more about the history of the people with whom she will be working. We take our seats in one of two auditoriums, part of a diverse crowd, 75 per cent Indigenous and 25 cent non-Indigenous. I feel exhilarated to be part of something destined to culminate in a historic re-writing of the national narrative and school textbooks, which have so far been devoid of details concerning the abuse, starvation, displacement, and murder of

Indigenous peoples. A few academics and poets have written about the deliberate extermination of the Beothuks in Newfoundland; periodic news reports appear on the subject of dilapidated housing, contaminated water, and high suicide rates on reserves; and, more recently, discordant notes have begun to surface about police brutality, in particular the habit of dropping intoxicated or homeless Indigenous males beyond city limits in mid-winter, where they freeze to death, and the ongoing saga of missing and murdered Indigenous women and girls.

The introduction by TRC chairman Justice Murray Sinclair sets a measured, if not exactly relaxed, tone for the proceedings. As he speaks, I can feel the collective blood pressure in the room drop. Helpers, trained to provide comfort and moral support to participants overcome by events and to those of us in the honoured, if unofficial, role of witnesses, line the walls with their supplies of water and facial tissues. A hush falls on the audience as the first few testimonies are shared, stories of physical and sexual abuse at the hands of nuns, priests, and residential school staff. One woman, for support, has brought her daughter and two sisters to sit with her on the stage, and a small dog that she holds and strokes in her lap, while slowly and with great difficulty, she recounts being incarcerated, constantly starved, beaten for speaking her own language, and deprived of the love and support of family.

The testimonies are shocking and heart-rending, all the more so because those who share them have such trouble getting the words out. All around me people are weeping. Facial tissues waft through the crowd, small white flags signalling, for many in the audience, surrender to power-ful feelings too long repressed. The official helpers collect used tissues in brown paper bags, which Justice Sinclair explains will be ritually burned later as a tribute to truth and to the intense emotions it evokes.

During the lunch break, Bronwen and I head across the street to the old Crystal Gardens, an art deco structure with curved metal and glass roof that has undergone various transitions over several decades, from swimming pool to arboretum and to its current incarnation as an overflow dining area for conference attendees who can't afford to dine in style at the Empress. We spot Joan Morris and her friends at a large round table and ask if we can join them. During the previous session, we'd heard Joan recount the story of her mother, admitted to the Nanaimo Indian Hospital at age eighteen—no one is certain why—in apparent good health, and not released until she was thirty-five, a physical and emotional basket case who demanded constant attention until her death. Seventeen years of so-called medical care leading to a ruined life.

Joan introduces us to her three friends. She is soft-spoken but direct, very open about herself, and curious to know about Bronwen's job. She also makes it clear when she learns I'm a writer that she is looking for someone to tell the story of Canada's segregated hospitals. In response to my question about her own time in the Nanaimo Indian Hospital, first in 1947 from age two to four, and then in 1951 from age five to seven, she gives a shorthand version of her two experiences there. She describes loneliness, boredom, physical and sexual abuse, restricted movement— thanks to being placed in a plaster cast from the waist down—mysterious injections, treatment with radioactive iodine, broken toes, removal of part of her lung, and doctors who stood around taking notes but did nothing to help. After her second stay at Nanaimo Indian Hospital, presumably cured, she was told she was going home, but was delivered instead by boat, at the tender age of seven, to the dock in front of Kuper Island Residential School, the looming Victorian edifice with its contingent of priests and nuns charged with the task of turning "savages" into good little Christians, whatever indignities this might require, or spitting them out broken, useless, and hell-bound.

After lunch, I thank Joan and promise to meet her the following week. Bronwen and I make our way to the session where clergy are to offer apologies for the role their denomination played in the physical, emotional, cultural, and sexual abuse of students in the residential schools. Anglican and United Church representatives do not hesitate to accept responsibility, making no attempt to justify or downplay what happened in their schools, or try to shift blame to the government. Then the Catholic representative steps forward, stating that all had been sweetness and light at the Port Alberni Residential School when he was in charge, the implication being that abuse in Catholic schools was rare and the case of a few misfits. A dozen or so people get up to leave. The audience erupts with angry shouts and denunciations.

"Bullshit."

"Tell the truth."

"Shame."

Scandal surrounding the Port Alberni Indian Residential School surfaced in the 1990s, when three Indigenous men, former students, went public with stories of sexual abuse at the hands of dormitory supervisor Arthur Henry Plint, who was eventually convicted and sentenced to eleven years in prison. *Stolen from Our Embrace* describes in detail the Willie Blackwater story, a moving account of this traumatic experience for one of the victims. The Catholic spokesman, visibly shaken, tries to continue his unapologetic apology and, once more drowned out by the response, sits down.

Exhausted by the tsunami of emotion that has washed over me, I leave for home on Thetis Island hoping to catch an early ferry. Bronwen stays for the second day of testimonies and is so overwhelmed by what she hears that she weeps all the way to the floatplane in the inner harbour, which is to take her back to Vancouver. She tells me by phone that among the hundreds of passers-by on the street the only person who acknowledges her distress and asks if he can help is an Indigenous man.

And so another journey has begun, this one closer to home but even deeper into the jungle of human emotions. I put down the phone. The tide is high now, my duplicitous sandbars submerged once again, only the ragged tips of firs on Penelakut Island still visible in the moonlight. I stand on the porch, a blanket pulled tight around my shoulders, and watch the shifting reflections in the water. In the distance, I can hear the faint sound of drumming.

two

Joanie, Kuper, and Nanaimo Indian Hospital _____

Joan Morris, or Joanie as she prefers to be called, is seated across from me at Ricky's Restaurant in a small plaza on Admirals Road, a major street that cuts the Songhees Reserve in half. Apparently, you don't argue with rank when it comes to colonial thoroughfares. She is spreading at least a hundred black-and-white photographs on the table, all associated with her mother's seventeen-year sojourn in the Nanaimo Indian Hospital, which operated from 1946 to 1967.

"That's my mother when she was admitted. She was healthy then. This is her a few years later, after the injections, bloated and sickly."

The difference is shocking. Confidence and youthful exuberance gone; and in their place a close-cropped woman with a puffy, unhealthy face and no light in her eyes. Joanie provides a running commentary on the photographs.

"This is Uncle Ivan, a patient at the same time, who almost died from a botched operation. That's the priest from Kuper who raped my friend. And this is the Nanaimo Indian Hospital where I was admitted at age two, and again at age five. I visited the place once after it closed to offer a prayer for those who died there. I'd never felt anything so cold before—it was like the hand of death of my neck."

As Joanie pauses over her coffee, I take a second look at the hospital's ramshackle wooden structure, faded and without character, a former army barracks that went from preparing youth for the killing fields in

Europe during World War II to providing medical short-shrift to Canada's Indigenous sick, administering forced sterilizations and gratuitous drug and surgical experiments. I'm shocked to notice the hospital's proximity and resemblance to the buildings at Vancouver Island University when it was called Malaspina College, where I'd often read my poems to classes taught by friends in the English Department.

Our second meeting takes place the following week at the Rebar Restaurant off Bastion Square, just up from the harbour in Victoria. I try to convince Joanie to order my favourite pot-stickers, but she turns up her nose at them, as well as at the house special, wheatgrass smoothies. She chooses fish tacos. While waiting to be served, we trade details of our dysfunctional backgrounds. Mine—poverty, a mother who died at thirty-five, and an alcoholic father—pales in comparison to what she's been through. It would be a gross understatement to say that Joanie was not welcomed into this world. Her injuries started as newborn when her mother tried to strangle her and managed to destroy one of her vocal cords. This explains why, despite our cramped quarters in the corner of the restaurant, I strain to decipher her words and why the nuns at the Kuper Island Residential School punished her so often for not speaking up.

Joanie's mother, Mary Theresa Morris, had wanted to be a nun, but was seduced and made pregnant, then forced into marriage by her parents. Her first child was aborted and no love was wasted on Joanie, the second. Sent to the Nanaimo Indian Hospital two weeks after Joanie was born, her mother ran away three times but was returned by the authorities. Eventually she came to view the hospital more as a place of refuge than a prison, a retreat where she could escape a marriage she did not want, a daughter she could not love, and the responsibilities that come with life on the outside.

In the Nanaimo Indian Hospital, time had stopped, meals were provided, a radio was allowed, if you were lucky, and a limited social network was close at hand. According to photographs, her mother's portion of the shared dorm was festooned with photos of friends and a large poster of Pat Boone, an indication that, despite being in her early thirties by then, she still saw herself as a teenager. As for Joanie's father, a member of the nearby Tsartlip tribe, she recalls being told that he'd been drinking at the time of her birth at her grandparents' house in Esquimalt. When awakened for the announcement, he raised himself on one elbow, saw the new arrival was a daughter, rolled over, and went back to sleep.

Joanie finishes her last fish taco, washes it down with water, and causally eyes my pot-stickers, while I wonder how she, as a religious person, manages to balance the forces of love and anger that must vie for ascendancy after what she's been through. She has plenty to resent in her personal and tribal history, grievances enough to drag any normal person to self-destructive behaviour, even suicide. On top of all that, she has recently been diagnosed with cancer. After so many negative experiences in hospitals, she has decided not to undergo surgery, requesting instead medication that will stabilize or slow down the disease. A recent biopsy to check out the progress of the cancer revealed small growths on her pancreas, which turned out to be benign. She has a lot of pain in the midriff area, she tells me, but tries not to let this affect her busy schedule. Joan is in demand in nursing circles, both as a spokesperson recounting her time at Nanaimo Indian Hospital and for her decades-long experience as a nurse's aide. Her interviews have not only been recorded on audio-tape and film, but are also the subject of the CBC documentary "State of Care" that aired on *The Current* in 2013. She has also, I notice, become an instant convert to pot-stickers, having decided that her new friend is not always wrong, at least when it comes restaurant food.

"Not bad," she says, with a mischievous grin, spearing another of those little satchels of succulence from my plate.

I am not surprised to find Joanie an enthusiastic eater, judging from her stories about rotten or inadequate rations at Kuper, a common theme among residential school survivors. As early as 1938, according to John Milloy in *A National Crime*, Inspector G.H. Barry described the deplorable conditions in the school:

> In the absence of some improvement in the variety and quantity of
> food served to the children at Kuper Island and the provision for a
> somewhat longer time for meals, I am somewhat apprehensive with

regard to the health of the pupils particularly those now stated to be infected with TB.[3]

Milloy sums up the situation across Canada, in which residential schools hired untrained staff to work in shoddy kitchen facilities, where the lack of cooking skills was surpassed only by a complete ignorance of nutrition. A report in 1946 found that the food "lacked sufficient amounts of vitamins A, B, and C." The children, moreover, received too little of nearly everything, including meat, and "not enough vegetables, whole grains, fruit, juices, milk, iodized salt and eggs."[4]

While staff ate well the students suffered, and the boldest or most desperate took to raiding the pantry late at night, or foraging amongst local farms. Malnourishment, if not outright starvation, was government policy. Complaints were ignored. The church-run schools, though purporting to adhere to the scriptural edict "Suffer the little children to come unto me" seemed to have reversed the procedure: "Let the children come to us and suffer." While agents and inspectors declared conditions a disgrace, hunger prevailed and the number of sick kids multiplied. When students or their families complained by post about school conditions, they were ignored. Deputy Superintendent of Indian Affairs, Duncan Campbell Scott, in one of his crasser moments, dismissed a child's formal complaint as an attempt to garner attention and ended with a telling comment that reveals either his total ignorance of conditions in the schools or his complete lack of concern: "Ninety-nine per cent of the Indian children at these schools are too fat."[5]

Our conversation at Rebar shifts back and forth between Joanie's injuries —her ruined vocal cord, the deliberately broken toes, early-onset diabetes— and her mother's eventual release from Nanaimo Indian hospital, after which she demanded to have all her meals served in bed. Obliged by tradition to look after her mom, Joanie was forced to abandon her ambition to be trained as a registered nurse.

Screwing up her face at the sight of a nearby diner chugalugging a whole glass of wheatgrass smoothie, Joanie alludes briefly to a murder at

29
-

the school on Penelakut, which I will learn about later from the victim's sister.

When I phoned a few weeks earlier to let Joanie know I was coming to Victoria and would like to spend as much time as possible interviewing her, she informed me she was going into the hospital but had not been told what for. Presumably it was a follow-up to her recent colonoscopy. I was surprised and startled that she had not demanded more information.

"Are you worried?" I asked.

"No," she said. "Last time I had a bad feeling when I went in for an operation, but not this time. I've been feeling that I'm ready to go home, but the Lord says my work here is not finished." Then she laughed, inquiring after my health.

As we wind down our time at the Rebar, where wheatgrass smoothies have been ignored and pot-stickers polished off, Joanie tells me that she was recently ordained. I don't understand her strong Christian faith after all her suffering at the hands of the Church. She knows I am not a believer and, though she refrains from overt efforts to restore me to the fold, insists she prays for me daily and makes a distinction between the loving Creator she knows and the so-called disciples who betrayed their calling.

"I want my people to know the love of God. That's the only thing that will heal them, restore their dignity."

three

Little Chatham, Saints, and Cod _____

"Shortly after I was born and my mother was shipped off to the Nanaimo Indian Hospital, I was living with my grandparents, Elizabeth and Andrew James, in Esquimalt Harbour. Grandmother was a midwife. Grandfather, a lovely man when sober, became violent and angry when drunk. He survived residential school on Penelakut Island but never talked about it. All that went to the grave with him. The house in Esquimalt burned down when someone knocked over a kerosene lantern. That's how we all came to be living with my great-grandparents, Tom and Alice James, on Chatham Island, my spiritual home."

Joan's and my latest culinary rendezvous takes place at the coffee shop at Oak Bay Marina, where offerings are limited but the view is unbeatable. The marina, with its vast flotilla of mostly unused sailboats and yachts, looks out at the snow-capped mountains of Washington's Olympic Peninsula and, more importantly today, at Little Chatham, or Tl'ches, the small outcrop of rock in the tumultuous Strait of Juan de Fuca south of Victoria, where Joanie spent some of the best years of her childhood in the loving of care elderly relatives. They survived on a diet of fruit and vegetables from their gardens, fish, clams, oysters, the occasional seal, and a variety of other creatures and marine plants unfamiliar to most non-Indigenous peoples. Grandfather Andrew, an avid fisherman, would sometimes paddle with Joan in the canoe from Chatham to the Songhees reserve in Esquimalt Harbour, some eight or ten kilometres in swift currents and very changeable

31

weather. He spoke little but conveyed a deep affection as he stopped regularly along the way to jig for cod and to show Joan how to bait a hook, offer a prayer of thanks for the catch, and put the fish quickly out of its misery with a sharp blow to the back of the head. Her great-grandmother, Alice, also known as Ts'emiykw', was the dominant presence on Chatham, the refuge Joan describes as an all-too-brief taste of "heaven on earth."

"Whenever I get lonely, I cry for the old ones," she confides over coffee and a chocolate muffin. "They were so loving. I never heard a harsh word, never knew hunger."

The old ones, including Granny Elizabeth, or Sellema, the closest to a saint Joanie has encountered in this mortal sphere, would tell her stories around the pot-belly stove on this remote and relatively treeless island, while winter storms raged.

"I never worried," she says. "They told me if the house caught fire or blew away in a storm, I should take refuge between two driftwood logs and that would keep me safe."

In one of our most touching moments together, she draws a circle on a flashcard I've brought along to make notes, writing great-grandmother Alice's name at the top, Granny Elizabeth on the left, Grandma Cecilia, who was blind from birth, on the right, and herself at the bottom alongside her closest friend Nancy Turner. A circle of affection, a circle of learning and healing.

Joanie has brought half a dozen large but fading photos that show her as a small child on Chatham, tending chickens with her great-grandmother. The old woman's ghostly image has almost disappeared from the photograph, sadly symbolic of the Songhees nation itself. The few sheep they raised provided wool to make knitted toques, gloves, and sweaters, to be bartered with the merchants in Victoria's Chinatown for the goods and produce they needed.

"Together we would all pick seaweed," Joanie says as we prepare to leave, "gather oysters, sea urchins, and something whose English name is chitons. They were the hardest to pull off the rocks."

"Not as hard to remove as the settlers," I can't resist adding.

Joanie nods her head and offers an indulgent smile. Life on Little Chatham was not easy, but it was a safe and caring environment for a child whose mother had rejected and almost killed her.

Not much remains of the settlement on Chatham, which looks like a barren rock in the distance. Boaters and picnickers have burned down the abandoned houses, but Joanie makes an annual pilgrimage there to commune with the spirits of her ancestors. By the early 1950s, the three Big Houses, where the community had come together for feasts, dances, and celebrations on neighbouring Discovery Island, were already long gone, the largest of the three islands having being declared a provincial park. Her small voice becomes even smaller as she reminisces about those times. I hope my portable recorder picks up what she is telling me over the noises of the coffee machines, loud conversations, and several small children screaming at their mothers for not giving them the delicious cookies and desserts maliciously located behind glass at a child's eye level.

As we leave, a small boy dashes out through the door ahead of us, shouting, "Where are the seals?" I tell him they're down by the floats, but to wait for his grandmother or nanny to take him there. It's a nostalgic moment not just for Joanie but also for me, as I remember bringing my own daughters here decades earlier after the seals had been released from Sealand. Instead of heading to an uncertain future in the open ocean, the seals opted to stay around the marina, cadging herring strips sold in the bait-and-tackle shop to curious tourists. My daughter Charlotte's favourite for its antics, including a clever backflip, was a plump, spotted female called Tea Bag.

I return the earlier batch of photographs, which I've scanned and placed in a leather-bound album so Joanie can keep them safe. I'm not expecting her question.

"What did you think after looking at all those pictures?"

She has something more than curiosity in mind, but I'm not sure what it is. I tell her the photos made me angry and upset at the waste of human lives, though I know it's also because old photos always remind me of my own losses and the relentless passing of time.

"This is just a drop in the whirlpool," Joanie says. "We've lost thousands, maybe millions."

I understand her use of the pronoun "we" to include the Indigenous peoples in the Americas, perhaps worldwide. She then talks about the

33

spread of smallpox blankets and of German-speaking doctors showing up at Kuper when she was there, with long needles to inject "medicines" into the chests of students, one of whom died shortly after.

I don't know how to respond to these stories. I've written about the long history of racism in Canada and read about medical experiments conducted by the US military on prison inmates, African-Americans and Hispanics, servicemen, veterans, foreign nationals, and other vulnerable groups. I'm also familiar with the infamous career of Dr. Donald Ewen Cameron in Canada, from his appointment as director of the Brandon Asylum to his cruel and destructive mind-altering experiments on psychiatric patients at the Allen Memorial Institute in Montreal. These experiments were part of MKULTRA, a brainwashing project funded by the CIA. Cameron had participated in the Nuremberg Tribunal in 1945, saving Rudolf Hess's life by declaring him insane. Then he headed the World Psychiatric Association, which had no shortage of former Nazi medics in its membership. When you go through the long list of illegal medical experiments conducted by the American, Japanese, German, and other military groups, you have to conclude that there is nothing we are incapable of inflicting on our fellow human beings, the more so if they are defenceless and seen as somehow inferior and, therefore, expendable.

Many Canadian historians dismiss Indigenous people's stories about smallpox and other deliberately introduced diseases as fabrications, arising from justifiable paranoia among peoples displaced, forcibly incarcerated, beaten, and sexually abused at the schools. I certainly don't dismiss those painful testimonies, so fresh in the minds of survivors, but I need more proof about smallpox and atrocities that occurred 150 years ago. It's an issue that will have to wait.

34

"I want to show you something," Joanie says, rescuing me from my confusing thoughts as we climb the steps to the marina's parking lot.

We take the waterfront route west along Dallas Road, driving past the golf course and waterfront homes of the wealthy, exquisitely located on

Songhees territory. Joanie is keen to show me her birthplace on a peninsula that extends into Esquimalt Harbour, with the ocean on three sides. The Songhees reserve lands are small, hemmed in by non-Indigenous housing, naval dockyards, and facilities, but the spot is a gem. A new First Nation wellness centre nearing completion dominates the entrance to the ocean-side of the reserve that leads down to the Big House and a scattering of private dwellings. Just past the construction site stands a sprawling, recently built one-storey complex in a fenced compound, intended as the administration centre for the Royal Canadian Navy's new submarine facility. I ask Joanie how it comes to be on Songhees land, already so small and crowded. She rolls her eyes, rubs thumb and forefinger together, and puts it down to dubious band politics, like the new row of townhouses encroaching on the reserve and the selling to developers of nearby Bear Mountain with its sacred ground.

We drive past the Big House, a gravelled parking lot, and some wild grass and trees on the few remaining acres of undeveloped land. Another house has been built on the site of Joanie's birthplace, the spot no longer available to her family. Instead, she lives in standard government housing on reserve land on the other side of Admirals Road, where most of the dwellings are identical, without character, and not built to last. She had to fight to keep that house when her mother died and pressure was put on her to leave. I wonder aloud who will staff the new wellness centre.

"Mostly non-Aboriginals," she says.

four

Say Uncle

Sandy Morris hooks onto a good-sized ling cod where a small ledge of rock extends out from the harbour. You have to be a local, or to have lost tackle on that jagged strip of sea-bottom, to know it's there, but the fish know and enjoy the protection and feed the reef provides. Not known as a fighter, the ling surprises Sandy with its fierce resistance. Perhaps he was not serious enough when he offered a prayer of thanks to the Creator, because the line breaks and Sandy loses his balance, falling backward in the boat. He expects to strike his head on the seat amidships, but awakens instead soaked from the exertion. He sits up in bed in the Nanaimo Indian Hospital, the dream receding, the hospital room coming slowly into focus. He must have dozed off during breakfast, a single half-eaten piece of toast on a plate encrusted with egg yolk. He pulls on his gown and slippers, anxious to find his brother Ivan, scheduled for lung surgery hours earlier.

He hurries to the dorm at the far end of the segregated hospital, the wood floors waxed and shining. Ivan's cot by the window is empty and stripped of its bedding. The timing of this ritual confuses Sandy, worries him. He races along the corridor to the station, where the duty nurse, on the phone and deep in conversation, does not acknowledge him. Farther along, outside the surgery, he spots two orderlies, leaning on their elbows across a trolley piled high with fresh linen, laughing.

"Where's my brother?"

The shorter of the two raises his eyebrows, in what could be irritation or bafflement at this brash young man who seems to have learned nothing from his time in the hospital.

He pushes Sandy in the chest, propelling him back into the arms of the second orderly. "Manners? You don't interrupt your superiors when they're talking."

"What's this?" The second man—Sandy thinks he recalls the name Joshua—holds him by the shoulders at arm's length. "Are you trying to assault me? I could report you to the director, but maybe some basic training is in order first." He grabs Sandy's left arm, twisting it behind his back and begins inching it upwards.

"He's too big for his britches," he says, giving the arm another tug. Sandy winces from the pain.

"You mean his loin-cloth." Both orderlies laugh.

"My brother." Sandy tries to speak, but the pain is too intense. His mouth remains open.

"You don't hear well, do you?" the first orderly whispers, pulling Sandy's ear. "What's that you say, your 'bother'?" His mouth so close Sandy can smell the stale gum and feel the warm breath. "You're the bother, you stupid savage!"

"Morris," Sandy tries again. "Ivan Morris." The orderlies exchange looks. The taller one, with the close-cropped, light-brown hair, retreats to the trolley, his stained green smock falling open to reveal a flaccid, hairless belly.

"Not much good he'll do you now. He's in the morgue," he says over his shoulder as he disappears into the medical supply closet.

Sandy's arm is released, but not before a final lift that sends him careening across the narrow corridor of the converted army barracks, where he lands on all fours.

The remaining orderly whistles at him as if summoning a dog.

Sandy races down the stairs two at a time, heart in his throat. It's dark in the morgue, and he has to feel his way along the wall for the light switch. He closes his eyes for a moment, not wanting his worst fear confirmed. But there it is, the solitary gurney. A white bed sheet carelessly tossed over the shape underneath, reaching almost to the floor on both sides, has failed to

37

cover the familiar feet. Sandy stands transfixed, a wave of nausea breaking over him. His limbs, reluctant to take the initiative, have to be coaxed into action. Once alongside the body, he runs his fingertips over the delicately formed toes. They are cold to the touch. Instinctively, he pulls the bed sheet over them, but the gesture serves only to uncover Ivan's face, eyelids closed in something deeper than sleep.

It's true, Sandy thinks. He's dead, my brother's dead. How can that be possible? How will I tell my parents?

A common procedure, they'd told him, the removal of a lung by cutting three to five ribs. He can still see the patronizing, matter-of-fact smile on the doctor's face.

He leans down for a moment to kiss his brother, his eyes welling with tears as the anxiety and terrible finality of the moment take hold. Unlike his feet, Ivan's cheek is still warm. Sandy shuts his eyes again, this time in prayer, but jumps back as a tickling sensation registers in his right ear. He leans over again, cheek brushing his brother's nose. A feather of breath. Sandy wants to shout, but is afraid of scaring his brother to death, this time permanently. Instead, he flings himself up the stairs and finds Flaccid Belly chatting with the duty nurse.

"He's alive, Ivan's alive!" Sandy gasps, his voice little more than a whisper. Annoyed by the interruption, the orderly tries to dismiss Sandy with a flick of the hand. Sandy looks around for the other tormentor, but he's nowhere to be seen. As he's about to ask the nurse to call a doctor, the orderly brushes him aside and strides off, his final words on the subject echoing down the long corridor.

"If you want your *bother* so badly, bring him up yourself."

Sandy's story takes on different configurations in my mind as Joanie and I watch a DVD, produced for teaching purposes by coastal health authorities. It contains two interviews, one with Joanie and one with her uncle, whose chosen name had been mistakenly heard and registered as "Sainty" by the nurse attending his birth. When she first recounted the experiences of Sandy and Ivan at the Nanaimo Indian Hospital, it struck me as just another example of the appalling treatment to which Indigenous peoples have been subjected by the medical profession and a racist society. Now, I see it as a moving tribute to their intense will to survive, to struggle not only against the perversity of individuals, but also against a system determined to exterminate or reduce to total subservience. Like the fiercely resistant ling cod, Ivan, too, beat the odds—the bungled operation, the medical neglect—by refusing to die. And his determined brother saved his life.

So many children did not make it out of the Nanaimo Indian Hospital alive, thanks to botched or unnecessary operations, drug experiments, neglect, abuse, and the absence of family. Conditions at the residential school and the Indian hospital had been so bad that Sandy, also diagnosed with tuberculosis, lost his own will to survive and felt that if he was going to die, he preferred to do it at home.

On his first escape attempt on December 30, 1953, Sandy was too weak to walk very far and returned to his hospital bed, his absence undetected. His fellow escapee asked when they'd make another try.

"Next year," Sandy said.

"What?" his friend cried, incredulous. "A whole year?"

"Well, it's only two days away," Sandy laughed.

The next attempt was successful and he ended up hiding for several months at the home of his aunt, who administered a drink made from a concoction of boiled bark that he was forced to imbibe daily in huge quantities, in lieu of water, tea, coffee, or pop. When he returned voluntarily to the hospital for x-rays, the results showed his tuberculosis was completely cured.

Sadly, after a troubled and alcoholic life, Sandy Morris is losing his memories to Alzheimer's disease, and his morgue rescue has been replaced by a residential school experience in which the priest discovers him and several friends keeping a stray pup alive under one of the outbuildings at the Kuper Island school and, for punishment, forces them to assist in drowning it.

Brother Ivan, recently deceased, had a long life, but with the inconvenience and discomfort of those three missing ribs.

Individual acts of violence, as painful as they are to learn about, pale beside the collective violence perpetrated on First Nations in Canada and

Indigenous peoples worldwide. Between the Conquest and the twentieth century, as many as 90 per cent of Indigenous peoples in the Americas were either murdered or died as a result of colonial violence and disease. Of those remaining, 40 per cent of the women were sterilized, and 40 to 60 per cent of the children forced into boarding schools did not survive.[6] A policy of assimilation or extermination, not as obvious but nevertheless insidious, continues to unfold in Canada, where poverty, displacement, humiliation, and deteriorating health and infrastructure have fuelled a sense of alienation, self-hatred, and hopelessness, causing an epidemic of suicides amongst the young in Indigenous communities.

In a documentary film called *The Canary Effect*, we're told, "it's hard for a leader in the United States to really acknowledge Indigenous pain because this brings up the whole cultural and historical legacy." In Canada it seems possible to acknowledge the pain and atrocity publicly, then do nothing about it. The official apology from the federal government in 2008, welcomed by many Canadians and a few survivors, has not been followed by the kind of praxis—turning words into action—that indicates honest intent. Instead, it was only lip service. While government lawyers accumulated fortunes in court opposing land claims and fair compensation for abuse, bureaucrats continued to issue thousands of oil and gas exploration leases on Indigenous land without consultation.

five

A Painful Diagnosis

Joanie's aunt Addie, from the Tsartlip First Nation in Brentwood Bay, lives in a small, subsidized, low-rise residential complex in Victoria, which I often passed when my former in-laws lived on Cedar Hill Road. She's a lovely, tender-hearted woman whose lifetime of health issues started at a young age with a serious case of tuberculosis of the bone. The only advantage this affliction afforded was to free her from the perils of residential school.

Well, not quite. Her life would be deeply scarred by the residential school experience of her parents and siblings, whose physical wounds and psychological bruises had turned some of them into abusers themselves. Although her tubercular leg was eventually cured and straightened by a bone graft, Addie's overall health continued to be at risk. She was treated badly by an alcoholic mother, abused by a brother, and sold by her father to men in Victoria's Chinatown. These confidences were not shared with any sense of rancor or blame, but out of a sadness for what a heartless colonial system had done to the family and community she loved.

What abuse wasn't meted out at home Addie found in abundance on buses, streets, and even in the hospitals. Dr. P must have forgotten his Hippocratic oath to do no harm when he said to her, "No wonder your health is so bad, you've let yourself become a tub of lard." And Dr. H, who refused to come near her but let his Asian assistant examine Addie, stood in the doorway and dismissed her complaints of back pain, black stools, and vomiting blood as "constipation." His treatment of Addie is a typical experience for many Indigenous patients, who are too often not taken seriously and assumed to be alcoholics, hypochondriacs, or malingerers. Because Dr. H's diagnosis remained on her charts, it became gospel, encouraging subsequent doctors to ignore Addie's recurrent nausea, which would later be properly attributed to double stomach ulcers.

A welcome relief from her loneliness and uncertain health was afforded by the presence of her grandson, a boy with attention deficit disorder, who lived with Addie for several years. Unfortunately, family stresses and shifting loyalties resulted in him being taken back to live with his parents, with no visiting privileges. Addie wept as she told me this.

Several hundred kilometres up the coast, conditions were equally perilous, as the Mounties rounded up children for the residential schools and segregated hospitals. Michael Dick's encounters with western-style medicine began in the so-called Preventorium, a tiny medical facility attached to St. Michael's Residential School in Alert Bay, where he was diagnosed with tuberculosis. He was taken to the Nanaimo Indian Hospital, where he was a patient twice, for a total of eight or nine years. Eventually hired to work at the same hospital, he would prove to be an observant and candid witness, confirming what I'd been learning from the experiences of Joanie Morris, her uncle Ivan, and her aunt Addie. As he tells Laurie Meijer Drees in the book *Healing Histories*, the procedures at Nanaimo Indian Hospital were often painful and done without sedation or painkillers:

> Reflecting on it now, I truly believe . . . there was a lot of medical pioneering going on . . .
>
> I knew, deep inside of me, what was wrong. But the whole process, the interaction was wrong. It wasn't about caring; the whole interaction between patients and staff wasn't about caring. It wasn't about that. The doctors and nurses were all hardcore Europeans. We heard so many racist comments. One of the orderlies, his last name was Krauss. He was in the Hitler ranks, and he made no bones about it! These were hardened people. There were lots of negative things. There were more negative aspects than there were positive to our time in the hospital.[7]

These "negative things"—in addition to boredom, loneliness, frustration, and racism—that Dick leaves to the reader's imagination suggest that the segregated hospital experience was often as bad or worse than the time spent in residential school. Many Canadians find it difficult to comprehend that deliberate medical experiments, abuse, and involuntary sterilizations could take place in a hospital environment, where care and healing are supposed to be the top priority. That difficulty, which I share, is fading as the testimonies accumulate.

In response to my efforts to articulate the links between the residential schools and segregated Indian hospitals, Suzanne Fournier, co-author of *Stolen from Our Embrace*, who knows as much as anyone about the impediments to good health amongst Indigenous peoples, offers this useful observation in an email:

> The TB hospitals worked hand-in-glove with the residential schools; they exchanged victims between their cold, dark and cruel mausoleums. The schools bred tuberculosis and a host of other, often fatal, diseases. Both institutions habitually sent aboriginal children home to die, victims of an utterly failed and depraved custodial conduct. I do remember being struck by how many people mentioned the TB hospitals too, as an equally painful imprisonment.

I have been hoping to meet Kim Recalma-Clutesi and her partner, Clan Chief Adam Dick, brother of the late Michael Dick mentioned above, at their home in Qualicum Bay on Vancouver Island. In my preparatory research, I chanced upon an article that appeared in the *Parksville Qualicum Beach News*, in which Kim—a filmmaker, former elected chief, and traditional knowledge keeper—is quoted as saying:

> My great uncle John died in the Port Alberni Indian Residential School on November 4, 1918. His cause of death was never recorded, his grave was never marked, he was never given a proper burial, his mother (my great grandmother), Agnes, was never informed of his death. He was only 14 years old. About 40 years ago, my late father-in-law, George Clutesi, told me of John's violent death. He was witness to John being beaten and thrown into the

43

root cellar for speaking his language and when the root cellar door was opened a couple days later; John had died from his injuries.

When I meet Kim, I am not expecting such a generous and vibrant welcome. A serious illness in the family has recently consumed much of her time and energy. My wife Ann and I are on a short holiday in Courtenay, a home exchange that enables us to kayak, cycle, and hike in familiar but for me unexplored territory. We arrive in Kim's driveway with kayaks strapped to the top of the car and receive warm hugs, a double blessing if you count the large, carved welcome figure presiding amongst the trees, and I do. Ann leaves to do some grocery shopping so I can talk privately with Kim.

Kim begins by telling me about Adam, who is out back doing a task in the carving shed. As a child, he was taken to live with his grandparents, well off the radar in remote Kingcome Inlet, to protect him from the perils of residential school. Spending much of their time in a dugout canoe, they would only take refuge in the village in the dead of winter when RCMP boats were not in the area.

"Four years old." Kim shakes her head. "Imagine how the separation and loneliness affected him. That was his parents' way of taking control, fighting back. He was being taught the structures of the culture and the clan system and stewardship, but at significant personal cost. Years later, when we watched the TRC report ceremony together on television, tears were running down Adam's face as he listened to the speeches. 'Until now,' he said, 'I never realized how lucky I was. Although I loved my grandparents and was safe, I was terribly lonely, no other children to play with.'"

It's a touching story and confirms not only Adam Dick's well-deserved reputation as a man of great knowledge and compassion, but also my impression of him from a video clip sent to me of Adam drumming and singing in Kwakwala at the pit-cook in honour of his eighty-seventh birthday. The clip ends with him offering a short translation of the message conveyed in his song, which highlights the difference between European and Indigenous views of the land and its precious resources: "We're not going to take it all; we're going to leave some for you."

I ask Kim about her early medical experiences.

"I spent a few months in the Nanaimo Indian hospital in the late '50s and '60s. I was four. My biggest memory is the physical and emotional brutality. No parents nearby. I remember Dr. Gamble, who was the head of Indian health. He scolded my mother for marrying my father, and said that my sickness was the result of the sin of marrying an Indian. Then he would say things to me like 'your parents have thrown you away.' What's so startling to recall is that we were put on experimental prophylactics for thirty years. You can imagine what that will do to your immune system. I started out with rheumatic fever and ended up with a form of rheumatoid arthritis in my teens and early twenties. When you're beaten down so much, you begin to believe it. The blame was put on the child: 'If you were a better person, you might not be as sick.'"

While Adam works in the carving shed, his and Kim's grand-nephew Weston, age two and a half, pushes his plastic wagon around the yard and back and forth on the deck. Kim talks with one ear cocked. As long as she can hear the sounds, she knows the little guy is okay.

"My folks started the RAVEN Society (Radio and Visual Education Network) in 1968 because there was no telephone service in any of the villages. My father who, along with his brother, was brutally abused at Kuper Island Residential School, understood the necessity of communication."

The two-way radio communication provided not only educational information and emergency contact, but also the opportunity for sharing stories and keeping in touch.

This contact was crucial, Kim explains, because "there had been a cloak of silence about everything in those days. People would talk about others, seldom about themselves. They were groomed for abuse and silence. My grandmother locked the door on all that. She was only a little girl when she suffered abuse. One day my mother got a call. I know it was in the early seventies, when I was a teenager. A woman was in distress. She'd gone into the hospital for a simple appendectomy and came out with her tubes tied. So my mother got on the phone and called Dr. Gamble, the head guy at the time. My mom was Icelandic. She'd lost her right to vote when she married my father and became a status Indian, but she watched what was happening closely. She was strong; she spoke out. She was very colourful, noisy. You had to be that way. She told Gamble he had no right to do that, that it was all part of the doctrine of discovery, the view that Indigenous people are savages, not human, and living in sin, which justified the violence, theft, and abuse.

"Unlike my father and other children at Kuper, I was never sodomized by a priest or tied to a cross and beaten with a stick. But there was plenty of abuse. And we were marched into the hospitals annually for head-to-toe x-rays. These things happened. Kids learned how to be invisible. My father was ferocious and worked hard to bring this all to the forefront. He also advised against payouts and suggested the money go instead into cultural restoration, languages."

Weston appears, face upturned, checking in, curious.

"Would you like an apple?" Kim asks.

He nods his head. "Affle."

He picks up a wedge, breaks off a piece, and gives it to me. When I pop it in my mouth, he offers another, then disappears to check on Papa (Grandpa) in the carving shed. I ask Kim how her negative medical experiences and those of her family have affected her feelings about the health-care system.

"I put my game face on," she says. "I listen to people's words, study their faces and body language carefully, and say what I need to say in order to make things happen. There's still so much racism in the system. I literally have to dance on the head of a pin to be a successful advocate. Without that, Adam would not have survived. It's not automatic, even today; Aboriginal people still have to fight for fair treatment. In Adam's case, the doctors refuse or delay treatment, hoping he'll die off. Let nature take its course, they say. He faces this constantly. They don't know who he is, or how important his life and work have been. Even without all that, he should be treated fairly and promptly. I call them the GQ boys [a reference to the men's fashion magazine, Gentlemen's Quarterly]. They have no cross-cultural awareness. I tell them what they're doing is culturally destructive, and rude. So they put a note on his chart saying his partner is showing signs of a split personality."

After some laughter, Kim talks about the challenges and impediments to good health care.

"We have to make personal connections with the health providers, then the right things get done. It's very difficult to go through this stuff, to be constantly humiliated. And Gamble, the man overseeing everything when I was young, the one who let it all happen, was always around, in the hospital, at our home, endearing himself to the family. You never felt safe. I think that's what abusers do. After they've done the grooming, they come back and do the visits. So you feel betrayed by your parents too, since they don't believe you. My sister died at sixty-three. The frequent head-to-toe x-rays and heavy meds she was subjected to in the '50s had something to do with that.

"There has to be a huge amount of counselling made available. Not the usual kind, as there are too many abusers still in the system. The trauma, personal or intergenerational, comes welling up. For a single woman with four kids, there's too much to deal with. She'll ask for counselling for her kids, but there is only money enough for one child. And it's too brief. There needs to be more counselling service available, because the trauma is perpetuated."

Weston is back, this time stuffing pieces of cheese into his great-auntie's mouth. Kim takes it all in stride and good humour. "We don't have a word for 'brat' in Kwak'wala, but we have every possible word for encouragement."

When he's gone exploring again, I tell Kim about my grandson Henry who, at the same age as Weston, was very interested in construction toys. As he walked down the street in Charlottesville, holding his father's hand, he noticed this elderly lady walking toward him. So he looked up at her and said, "Have you seen my front-end loader?"

Kim laughs and offers a story to match mine. "I was changing Weston about a month ago and I picked up this pair of clean pants which weren't quite dry. 'Darn it,' I said. So, Weston, in his gentle, little voice, replies, 'O fuck, that too bad.' Around a lot of adults obviously, but at least he used the word correctly."

I'm interested in Kim's thoughts about what needs to be done and ask how my own project might be of some use.

"We grew up in a time when the horrors were unspoken," she says, "but my mother did not grow up in that and she questioned what was happening. She spoke about the mass sterilization going on. Canadians don't know that the Nanaimo Indian Hospital was used for mass sterilization. I think getting the story out is a good thing, but it's not for everybody."

I ask her to explain.

"You know, we have a ritual ceremony called *degita*, during which you wash away things that don't belong to you, such as an accident, some big pain, a serious offence. When this takes place, as Adam says in his eloquent speeches, you don't look back. I think the problem with the some of the Truth and Reconciliation process is that it becomes a way of re-opening the wound, continually peeling the scab off. People get stuck in the story. The story has to be set at the beginning point. You don't just leave people hanging out there. There's an oddly satisfying thing that happens with some of the people who just sit and listen. It doesn't heal the churches to have their members sitting there crying alongside the victim. It's insulting actually. They need to get down in the trenches and work for the people, with the people, try to assist in some real change."

I'm not sure I understand what Kim is getting at here, but don't want to interrupt for clarification. However, it reminds me of German playwright Bertolt Brecht's alienation theory, in which he rejects the notion of theatrical catharsis, which gives people an emotional jag but leaves them capable of returning unchanged the next morning to their jobs at the concentration camp. What he wanted was theatre that disturbs people, challenges their assumptions, makes them want to hang around afterward and debate the issues presented on stage. In other words, shedding a tear is not necessarily the first step towards action, especially the change that is needed. The word "praxis" comes to mind again, feelings or ideas that result in action, an official apology that is not just lip service but brings about positive change.

However, Kim is quick to elaborate. She's talking about victims, not perpetrators.

"I'm thrilled with how the TRC reports have been laid out, but I'm not thrilled with how people have been left with their stories dangling. And I don't like how they've been left with their addictions and suicidal thoughts, their self-loathing. I think people have been left with their lives interrupted. Some of the crew on my dad's fish-boat said that when they spent their compensation money, they felt cheapened, as if they'd been paid a fee for services rendered, however involuntarily. It's not enough to have bits of counselling that never last long. The horrors are still there, the self-loathing. My father argued for the compensation to go for cultural restoration, invest that money in restoring land, languages, dignity. The TRC hearings may serve other people or a political process, but they don't necessarily serve the person against whom a crime has been committed."

Now I understand. Of the three men who first testified against their abuser at Port Alberni Residential School, and helped set the whole process in motion, one took his own life shortly thereafter. This should have been a lesson for us all.

"I think the story has to be told," Kim says. "I don't think people know about medical experiments. My father was one of those who had the big needles stuck in his chest at Kuper Island. Medical records aren't available anymore. There was a lot of cleansing of Indian affairs documents, reports removed. People I know working for Indian Affairs in small communities were ordered to burn documents. We need to be very clear that the bureaucracy of the day, those working for Indian Affairs and Health Canada, were very conflicted, and those destructive policies are still being executed today. People are being demonized, demoralized, sterilized. How can you do those things and sleep at night? I think as a country we have to grow up and own it. Not just what happened with the TRC—that was needed—but enough now with people having to recite and repeat their stories. Enough."

Weston is not responding to Kim's call, so she disappears to the backyard and carving shed to look for him. I go in the other direction and find him playing with the tiny fountain on the porch, stirring the water with a bent stick. Kim finds us, smiles, and gives him a compliment and a big hug.

"There is this monstrous distrust of the medical and political system. It's not enough for Murray Sinclair to say it; the politicians have to say it, the government of the day has to say it. And that's where Justin Trudeau has been incredible. He's the only one to admit there were atrocities. But his bureaucracy has to respond accordingly. At the end of the day, nothing has changed yet in Indian land. They've got to stop saying to the United Nations that we're okay, that Canada's human rights record is good, that our children are protected."

Without pausing, Kim launches into an anecdote about requesting funding from a couple of religious foundations, which had been set up to encourage healing, to help her create a series of books for children about the gathering and preparing of traditional foods, to teach them about husbandry, working with and caring for the environment, about responsibility and sharing. Both committees turned her down because they could not see how this would engage with their congregations. Kim exploded.

49

"What does this have to do with your congregation? Obviously, the healing is not for us. This is a healing fund for your guilt, for god's sake. It has nothing to do with trying to right the wrongs."

When funds are set up, she explains, "there can't be some sort of Kumbaya moment for everyone to sit there and cry and feel better, a kind of voyeurism that makes our people feel like monkeys. If we're going to heal, the churches have to do more than have a speaker once a year."

"You mean for their annual emotional jag?"

"Exactly, and I'm the usual suspect."

This has been such a rich sharing experience, I'm reluctant to admit that our time is running out. We talk briefly about Duncan Campbell Scott, the *eminence grise* behind the residential schools.

"He was the guy that did all the prohibition legislation. An odd man, he wrote poems about the vanishing noble savages," Kim says, "and then made it happen legislatively."

I mention Pierre Trudeau's famous White Paper, which proposed abolishing the Indian Act on the grounds that no group of Canadians should have special status. Kim tells me that her late father, who was part N'isga'a, was involved in fighting on behalf of the Calder case when the Supreme Court came down on the side of the N'isga'a. He was sitting with members of his family in the prime minister's office when Pierre Trudeau apologized, saying, "I got it totally wrong."

After reminding me that a change in deputy ministers and senior bureaucrats will be needed for any serious improvement to take place, Kim chats with me about traditional foods, about working with her friend and collaborator, ethno-botanist Nancy Turner. I mention that my wife Ann studied with Nancy years ago and, partially as a result of taking the course, named her daughter Camas.

Right on cue, the car swings into the driveway, Ann waving as she negotiates a turn, the vehicle and two kayaks strapped on top only briefly obscuring the white, carved figure and its continuing message of welcome.

six

The Cornerstone of Belief _____

Before ocean levels began to rise again, after the glaciers receded, Thetis and Penelakut were one island attached by a saltwater marsh and part of a group now known as the Gulf Islands, a short ferry ride from the city of Chemainus on Vancouver Island. Some of my neighbours take comfort in thinking the inhabitants of Penelakut Island never lived on Thetis, but for anyone with eyes to see, every major beach on Thetis contains deep layers of shell midden, indicating centuries, if not millennia, of harvesting clams and oysters and of undeniable habitation by the Penelakut, as they now officially call themselves and their island.

When British warships appeared on the scene, flexing imperial muscles, they decimated villages and forced the removal or amalgamation of communities. Then settlers arrived, who wanted the north island for themselves, and finally commercial fishermen, who demanded a deeper channel to access the safe anchorage of Telegraph Harbour and made surgical separation inevitable by dredging. The resulting Cut, as it was called post-op, turned out not to be Shakespeare's "unkindest cut of all," because both sets of islanders found it useful if, at times, divisive.

I was vaguely aware of the existence of Kuper Island Residential School—whose acronym, KIRS, sounds appropriately like the word "curse"—and its sordid record of physical and sexual abuse before I met Joanie. However, when she told me she'd been a student at that school it all took on a more personal note, the travesties happening to a friend and only a few hundred yards from the house I now inhabit. I'd seen the documentary film made in 1997 by Gumboot Productions, for which my friend Penny Joy was Associate Producer. As a single mom and a recent immigrant from the UK, Penny had spent a couple of years in a gestalt commune at the south end of Penelakut Island, long before most First Nations began to re-assert their rights to land, respect, and self-government. So, it must have been a shock to her as well to hear the painful testimonies emerge, piecemeal, from survivors gathered for the healing ceremony.

Joanie and I are sitting in the living room of number 5 Cooper Street, a house in a spacious yard on the Songhees reserve in Victoria that is used for counselling. I've invited her to watch *Return to the Healing Circle* with me, knowing it will bring back a lot of memories. The film opens with a blunt statement by James Charley, a survivor of abuse at Kuper Island Residential School, about the violent deaths of eight of his residential school friends, from car accidents, slashed wrists, drug overdoses. All of them were victims of sexual abuse by the religious priests and Brothers of the Missionary Oblates of Mary Immaculate.

This is followed by a close-up of the school's cornerstone. Begun as a trade school in 1890, the Kuper Island Indian Residential School did not close until the late 1970s. Almost a hundred years of misery, affecting five generations. The brick building whose demolition is being celebrated was opened in 1914, the same year that initiated a slaughter on the battlefields of Europe. The granite slab sits on the edge of the pier. Various survivors begin to share their experiences, including Bill Seward, who remembers being beaten for speaking his own language, forced to kneel in a corner for hours reciting Christian prayers, only to be beaten again each time he stopped. No one explained why he couldn't speak his own language, when English-speaking Christians were going about their peculiar devotions using Latin.

"Delmar!" Joanie is half out of her chair, recognizing one of the survivors who has just appeared on the screen. "I gave talks with him a few years ago about the residential schools and Indian hospitals."

A gifted artist and admired leader, Delmar Johnnie admits his discomfort over the return to Penelakut as an adult: "All my memories are connected with the child that lived here. I prayed I'd be strong enough to face all these feelings." As the camera follows Delmar into the school gym, where punishment and abuse by the staff were not uncommon sports, Joanie covers her face and releases something between a moan and a sigh.

"After all my preparations for coming," Delmar continues, "I had not expected to feel all this. That six-year-old child had no reason to be here. Didn't deserve that. No child that age deserves to be pushed around like that. I hated it. Lots of sorrow because I was no longer a kid." He pauses a moment, then begins to speak again, his voice shaky. "Drinking was how I handled it. There's more to healing than just to stop drinking. I had to look back at that stuff and deal with it."

Another sequence shows Delmar standing outside the sweat lodge, an eagle feather in his hand. He's offering a group of young men a parable about the eagle feather which, when rubbed the wrong way, looks beaten and frazzled, but brushed the right way has its beauty and usefulness restored.

One of the most touching scenes in the film takes place between James Charley and his brother Tony, who speaks of his twenty wasted years of denial, refusing to talk about the sexual abuse both he and his brother endured at the school.

"Those people were hypocrites of the worst kind," Tony confides. "I couldn't understand what they were doing. I thought maybe that's what it means to be a Christian."

He recalls the significance of numbers, used instead of names in the school, how no one could relax in the playing fields until the Brother on the fourth floor blew a whistle and called out a number. When the unlucky boy whose number had been called went to entertain the Brother for the afternoon, you could relax. You knew you were safe. Giving a child a number, instead of a name, made him or her less than human, and easier to abuse.

James looks at his brother and nods. "I'm forty, you're forty-two. Where have we been for the last twenty-five years? That's what the church done. They set out to divide us. And they done a pretty damn good job."

"We could have been good support to one another," Tony says.

The film ends where it began, with the camera focused on the residential school cornerstone on the edge of the pier. As the music builds, the stone is nudged off its perch and plunges into the ocean, its flat side

53

sending a huge plume of water into the air. Those gathered on the dock cheer, salt water and tears streaming down their faces. As the ripples spread outward, a message of resistance and renewal moves across the surface toward Thetis Island and beyond and a downpour of rose petals descends on the glistening waters of Telegraph Harbour, each in remembrance of a loved one lost or a life destroyed.

It's against this background that Joanie refers again to the murder of Richard Thomas at the Kuper Island Residential School, but advises me to get the full story from his sister Belvie Brebber, who appears in the film and now lives in the city of Duncan, a Vancouver Island community once made up of remittance men and other colonial misfits, but now a thriving multicultural community, in which the Cowichan people figure prominently. I promise to do that and take my leave of Joanie and her troubling memories.

Boat traffic in Canoe Pass picks up as the tide rises to midway, kayaks first, followed by aluminum skiffs and smaller outboard runabouts, then at full tide an assortment of larger craft, including medium-sized sailboats with six feet or less of draft. I enjoy the distraction this traffic provides in summer, another reminder of the pleasure and comfort to be found in the daily and seasonal rhythms of living on the coast, huge bodies of salt water filling and emptying harbours and long inlets, bringing with them driftwood, stray boom-logs, and a variety of natural and man-made flotsam. While the pass experiences extremes of high and low tides, it's sufficiently protected that none of the violent storms are felt here, except for the occasional collapse of a wind-blown tree.

Although this landscape of mountains and sea with its ten thousand miles of ragged coastline is dramatic, the product of countless millennia of glacial carving, volcanic action, erosion, and the slow but relentless shifting of continental plates, the climate and living conditions of the inner coast have been challenging but relatively benign for centuries, with abundant seafood and animals, disturbed only by the occasional raiding party or territorial dispute. The arrival of Europeans changed all that. Within a century, the original population of the coast had been decimated by greed,

54

disease, and racist assumptions of moral, cultural, and intellectual superiority. Another few decades and the sea would be devastated, the salmon gone, and the whales that depended on them topping the endangered species list.

This evening there's a youth from one of Thetis's religious camps casually propelling his stand-on paddleboard past my place, wearing a bathing suit but no lifejacket. Still young enough to claim membership amongst the immortals, he's untroubled by thoughts of death by drowning or by the sad history of Penelakut Island, relishing only the moment and a body that cleans and repairs itself without fuss. I remember those days fondly and am glad for him.

seven

Belvie, Richard, and the Holy Brothers _____

Belvie Brebber, another of Joanie's friends and a survivor of both Kuper Island Residential School and the Nanaimo Indian Hospital, is not up when I drive to her place in Duncan, the only pink cottage on the Cowichan reserve, whose separate administration buildings and Big House I'd passed on the way out of town. The Duncan band is one of seven tribes comprising the Cowichan Nation, Hul'q'umi'num' speakers, the largest Indigenous group in British Columbia. All the curtains are drawn and there's no response to my light tap on the door. Just as well, as I don't want to say hello and immediately have to ask if I can use the bathroom. I slip into the car and head back to the tiny downtown, where I find a restaurant, order a decaf, two regular lattés, and some blueberry muffins to go. When I return to the reserve, one curtain in the kitchen has been drawn back, so I know Belvie is up. Already warming her hands around a mug of homemade coffee at the door, she invites me in and says she'll tackle the lattés and muffins later.

I have a number of questions in mind for Belvie, including her traumatic experiences at the Nanaimo Indian Hospital. We talk a bit about Joanie, whom Belvie knew as a child in the hospital and also at Kuper Island Residential School. She is relaxed and does not seem the least bit uncomfortable talking about intimate events in her life or the more general subject of racism.

"Sometimes it's so subtle," Belvie says, sipping her coffee, "that you hardly notice. You wonder what it's all about, then the light goes on."

She tells me about a recent visit to a Duncan pharmacy, where she went to the counter with forty dollars worth of merchandise, only to be told by the clerk that debit cards were not accepted.

"I said, 'Why not, I've used mine here and every other store in Duncan accepts them.'" The woman obviously had her own notions about the ability of "Indians" to pay for their purchases. Fortunately, the manager overheard the exchange, stepped in, apologized for the "misunderstanding," and completed the transaction.

Our conversation ranges widely, always coming back to the residential school, where abuse and trauma dominated the curriculum. She speaks matter-of-factly about the sexual abuse at Kuper, about being told to take some dirty linen to the laundry room, a dark, scary region in the basement. She was reluctant to go, and several girls offered to take her place, but the Mother Superior said, "She has to learn sooner or later. Let her go." The light switch did not work in the laundry room, but she could vaguely see the machine at the end of the room and thought she could toss the clothes on top and quickly retreat. That's when a shape emerged from the shadows. She tried to make a dash for the door, but was grabbed by the ankle and fell, banging her head on the floor.

"Did you see who your attacker was?"

"Yes," she says, offering the Father's name. I ask whether the nuns or the Mother Superior ever assisted in the sexual abuse, other than the obvious pimping Belvie has hinted at.

"No," she says. "We called her The Destroyer. Her task was to break our spirits and she did an excellent job of that."

On another occasion, the same Father appeared at her bedside at night, waking her up with the excuse that he needed to talk to her about her younger sibling Richard, who, he said, was very sick. When Belvie rose groggily and followed him between the rows of sleeping girls, the Father cautioned her in a whisper not to make a sound. However, the Mother Superior, whose door was ajar, demanded in a loud voice to know who was there.

"It's me," he whispered. "I heard a noise and thought one of the boys might be on the prowl. Go back to sleep."

Belvie was then ushered into the infirmary and held down, a large hand across her mouth and nose, so she could hardly breathe, never mind scream. She passed out and regained consciousness later to find herself naked on a bed of towels, her pyjamas lying on the floor. Gathering her things, she retreated to the bathroom, where she sat for a while, obsessing over the fact that everything looked unfamiliar. Eventually, she realized that she'd been viewing it for the first time from a different perspective.

I point out the strangeness of what she's just said, the fact that, having just been raped, she was focussing on something entirely unrelated, as if her body were assisting in the denial of what had happened. I mention a scene in the movie version of Ambrose Bierce's short story, "Incident at Owl Creek Bridge," where the soldier about to be hanged finds himself concentrating instead on the movements of a caterpillar crossing a leaf.

Belvie ponders her coffee for a moment. "I developed that technique at the Indian hospital," she says. "I was able to avoid a lot of pain by making my mind go elsewhere."

Belvie talks about the other side of the Father who raped her, how popular he was with the students, who hung on his every word. "He was like a father figure for all of us. He called me Sparky, because I always had a twinkle in my eye when there was a family visit or some outing planned. But after he had his way with you, he dropped you flat."

Belvie's brother, Richard Thomas, had never been sick, although any kind of ailment, even tuberculosis, would have been a better fate for this intelligent and sensitive young man who'd dreamed of becoming a priest.

"He'd have made a wonderful one, too," Joanie assured me on our previous visit.

I had a rough idea of what had happened to Richard from what Joan told me, but I wanted to hear Belvie's version of events.

Having reached leaving age for residential school students, Richard had phoned home from the Kuper Island Residential School on Wednesday to talk to his mother, and then to his older sister Belvie, who was no longer at Kuper. He was in high spirits about his grad party on Friday.

"You know, Belvie," he said, his voice altered, "when I get out of this hellhole I'm going to tell everything." That's when Belvie heard a click and the phone went dead.

The next evening Richard was found hanging by the neck in the gymnasium. The students were forced to walk past his body, and the Brother warned them that this is what could happen to people who talk too much. When I requested a copy of the death certificate from the provincial government, I noticed that his death was attributed to "strangulation," rather than "hanging." However, in the section for the cause of violent death, the boxes indicating "accident" or "homicide" remain empty, but the box for "suicide" is marked with an X. There's something else suspicious about this official certificate: the date of death. The month of June and the year 1966 are clearly typed, but the day has been changed by hand to the 2nd, which may indicate a discrepancy between the coroner's assessed time of death and the one finally reported. To my eye, magnifying the page, it seems as if the original typed date was the 1st of June, as the horizontal line of a typed "t" is still evident, along with the vertical shaft of the number one. Was this simply the correction of a typographical error or a deliberate alteration demanded by the authorities? It might be an indication that the medical examination showed Richard Thomas died on June 1, the day of the phone call home, but that he was declared dead by the authorities when "found" hanging in the gym on the morning of June 2.

"When we were walking back from the graveyard days later—Mom and my sister and I—we were a few steps behind the Brother we think was responsible. Mom called to him three times, but he did not respond. After the fourth time, he turned around and, in a loud, threatening voice, demanded, 'What do you want?' Mom was so shocked we had to hold her up. She whispered, 'Brother, if you know anything about my son's death, please tell me.' That's when he turned his full wrath on her, bellowing that she already knew everything he had to say on the subject."

"Do you think he killed Richard?" I can't help putting the question bluntly.

Belvie looks up at the television for a moment, where a muted meteorologist is predicting the weather.

"Some years later," she says, "I wrote a twelve-page letter to the Brother, who'd been promoted to the priesthood by then and was working closely with the bishop in Victoria. I took the letter to the St. Andrew's Cathedral. He was not there that day, so I asked one of the clergy to give it to him."

"Did he respond?"

"No. Two days later, he apparently left the city. Sent to the Yukon, I think."

"Did you make a copy of the letter?"

"No. I thought of that later. I think I still have some of the notes I made."

"Has he ever been charged?" Belvie shakes her head slowly.

I make a mental note to ask her about the contents of the letter. The clergyman we're talking about is already familiar to me, a man whose name has come up more than once in connection with sexual abuse. Then, I surprise her with a white 8.5 x 11-inch sheet of paper on which I've typed his name, address, and phone number. "He's living in one of Vancouver's poshest districts, in a Catholic retirement home."

Belvie looks as if she's seen a ghost. "Are you sure it's him?"

"I found the information online, Canada411."

"None of us believed it was a suicide. A few years ago, one of the men in our community told me confidentially that he and some friends were playing behind the gymnasium the night before Richard's body was found. They heard some commotion and saw the priest and Brothers carrying something heavy wrapped in a blanket to the gym, but hid so they wouldn't be noticed and did not investigate."

I ask Belvie how she feels about this, and whether charges should be brought against him.

"He'll be in his late eighties by now," she speculates, glancing at the images on the large television screen that dominates the small room. A nasty-looking type is making threatening gestures to someone off-camera. "The government, Church, and police will protect him. And the lawyers would make mincemeat of me."

"A lot of shit will hit the fan, of course," I reply, "but the Catholic Church is under pressure to make amends and try to regain the enormous amount of respect it's lost over the last couple of decades. The question is whether you have the will and strength to go through with a trial. Think about it. We can discuss it another time."

Several months go by before I have a chance to talk to Belvie about her experience at the Nanaimo Indian hospital, where she was raped by an orderly at age five, while encased in a full-body cast, then locked away in a closet by a nurse determined to break her spirit. That's when she'll recall, as well, her friend Margaret Pelkey being raped at Kuper Island Residential School. Because she subsequently refused to obey any of the rules, avoiding classes and dancing wildly in the schoolyard, the staff sent Margaret to Riverview Hospital in Coquitlam, the mental asylum previously known as Essondale, where fifteen more years of her life would be wasted.

I give Belvie a hug and reach for the door handle, but turn back to ask, "Is there any hope for change? Do you see signs of improvement for Indigenous people?" I'm thinking of the racist incident in the pharmacy.

Belvie wipes her eyes again. "Yes, when I see the young people I worked with in the drug and alcohol program getting educated and going into the professions, it makes me happy."

eight

Experimental Bodies _____

I magine looking around for starving or malnourished individuals, not
so you can provide them with enough food to regain their health and
strength, but because they are ideal guinea pigs for experiments you have
in mind. Sound familiar? It should, as it's the plot or sub-plot, not only for
real-life events, but also for a few books and movies set in concentration
camps or out-of-the-way places worldwide: Japanese doctors performing
medical experiments on Korean prisoners during the Occupation; Josef
Mengele and other German doctors doing tests on Jews, twins, homosexuals, communists, Roma, and other "undesirables" during World War II;
American doctors failing to treat African-American sharecroppers who
had syphilis in order to conduct a forty-year study of its "natural" progress; or the brainwashing experiments on helpless psychiatric patients in a
program called MKULTRA at the Allen Memorial Institute in Montreal,
where Dr. Ewen Cameron, with support from the CIA, subjected patients
to LSD, excessive shock treatments, sensory deprivation, and severe condi-
tioning, all in the interests of US military intelligence.

Given the damage done in residential schools, it should hardly be sur-
prising to discover that nutritional experiments and deliberate starvation
were in keeping with the overall vision of government and Indian Affairs.
All this is going through my mind as I drive through pelting rain towards
Port Alberni, a remote fishing and logging community on the west coast of
Vancouver Island. Most of the best timber and old-growth forest has been

clear-cut by the lumber barons—MacMillan Bloedel, Weyerhaeuser, and their ilk—who skinned the landscape and left a tiny park called Cathedral Grove to remind us all of what has been lost. Port Alberni's only significance for me, other than a pit-stop en route to the beaches of Tofino and Ucluelet, is the great earthquake of March 28, 1964, which sent a tidal wave up Alberni Inlet, devastating the town. My uncle Art Bates, who ran British Motor Products in Vancouver, told me he'd acquired a nearly new Austin-Healey sports car from the insurance company for next to nothing because it had been swamped during that massive influx of salt water. I am heading toward another kind of tsunami, this one having to do with experiments on undernourished children at Port Alberni Indian Residential School, one of six residential schools, a.k.a. laboratories, across Canada during the 1940s and 1950s. News of these infamous experiments has recently swept through the newspapers and social media, sixty years after the fact, and is creating an uproar in this particular community amongst survivors.

I find a spot in the parking lot of the Tseshaht gymnasium and make my way into the crowded space, past the registration desk and tables stacked with promotional material. On the wall behind the microphone, a quotation from Nelson Mandela catches my eye, one that addresses the widespread feelings of inadequacy surrounding the Canadian government's official apology to First Nations: "True reconciliation does not consist in merely forgetting the past. Reconciliation means working together to correct the legacy of past injustice."

As the ceremonies begin, there is a rattle-song by performers in headbands and red Tseshaht t-shirts, followed by drumming, during which a line of women stand with hands open, palms upward in the traditional welcoming gesture.

"The government failed us," Chief Braker says, "but we're growing again, physically, spiritually. We're gathered here with no government funding. We thought the full story had come out, but that was not true, as we learned in June when Dr. Mosby's article appeared."

The revelation in question is Ian Mosby's disclosure, which went viral on social media before hitting the news, that nutritional experiments were conducted on Indigenous children in six residential schools across the country, including the one in Port Alberni. People gathered tonight by the Nuu-chah-nulth Tribal Council include journalists, health-care workers, and former residential school students and their relatives, many of whom have come from great distances to have their flood of questions answered.

Chief Braker condemns the government not only for allowing the children to be used as guinea pigs, but also for its failure to alert the families involved even as the results were being callously published by the Canadian Medical Association. His speech, which includes a list of recommendations to the government, draws thunderous applause from the audience. When Mosby is introduced and begins to talk, the rumble of voices in the gymnasium falls silent. People lean forward in their seats, even the elderly woman seated nearby in her wheelchair. She places her arthritic hands for comfort on the knees of two grandchildren, a boy and a girl on either side. Mosby, a postdoctoral fellow at McMaster University and a historian of food, health, and nutrition, graciously acknowledges his surprise at the attention his research has received. To his credit, he admits that the general information about the nutritional experiments was first released by Health Canada and reported in the *Vancouver Sun* on April 26, 2000, thirteen years earlier, but had been hardly noticed at the time. His timing and additional research, producing the necessary names and details at a moment when Indigenous issues are very much in the news, has produced the desired effect.

He speaks of Dr. Lionel Bradley Pett who, in 1952, oversaw the use of a certain kind of white flour that was tested on residential school students in Newfoundland and St. Mary's Indian Residential School in Kenora, Ontario. He explains the proposed rationale, then zeroes in on the experiments at Port Alberni Indian Residential School, where Dr. Percy Moore, superintendent of Medical Services, Indian Affairs—at that time a branch of the Department of Mines and Resources—conducted experiments, keeping the students malnourished, their diets lacking almost all vitamins, and giving milk only to a control group. As Mosby goes through the roster of affected residential schools, including St. Mary's, Shubenacadie, Cecilia Jeffrey, Norway House, and Spanish Hills, I recall his written observation that this amounted to "a brazen case of social engineering" that can only happen in a climate of systemic racism. Mosby's article on the topic, which was published in 2013, describes the involuntary experiments as examples of "exploitation and neglect" that violate "the Nuremberg code of experimental research ethics."[8]

As the details unfold, anger mounts in the audience. Individuals who have only heard about the experiments through radio, TV, or newspaper accounts begin to line up at the microphones to vent their anger and share their own residential school experiences of deprivation and neglect. Deb Foxcroft, president of the tribal council and daughter of the late James Gallic, a former student at Port Alberni Residential School, sets the tone by recalling her father's description of the school as a prison and saying that "the cows and pigs ate better than students did." Not having had that experience, she finds it difficult at first to believe the government would deliberately allow children to go hungry.

"What can I do," she asks, "to assist my people to heal?"

Medical experiments on unsuspecting patients ought to be common knowledge these days, with the exposure by John Marks and others of larger-scale projects such as MKULTRA and Project Paperclip, the latter providing immunity for Nazi medical scientists in exchange for their knowledge and participation in US chemical warfare experiments. With seemingly innocuous code names such as Project Bluebird (later, changed to Artichoke), Project Chatter, Operation Plumbob, and Project Chariot, these experiments involved the use of truth serums, testing the effects of nuclear fallout on unsuspecting soldiers and civilians, including the Inupiaq band of Point Hope, Alaska, in 1958. The subjects of these clinical trials were often selected based on gender, and included hospital patients, prison inmates, the poor, and the racially disenfranchised.

Canada was a destination of choice for some of these experiments. US military dispersed toxic clouds of cadmium over Winnipeg and several American cities to test its effects on the human respiratory system. Before his period at the Montreal Neurological Institute, Ewen Cameron conducted experiments on mental patients at Brandon Mental Health Centre. He forced some to be exposed naked to highly intense heat lamps for extended periods, or kept them in electric cages that overheated the body and induced comas. Others were injected with large doses of insulin. Without proper oversight, vulnerable populations will always be exploited

65

by the ruthless elements in a society, usually with government approval. Now many similar experiments are done overseas as a result of bribes paid to unscrupulous officials.

The next speaker is brief, insisting that residential school taught him to hate himself and everything else. Then Margaret, who worked for a lawyer involved in the flawed residential school compensation process, speaks of not being able to have children. She became pregnant and delivered a child at residential school, but never knew what happened to it and what might have been done to her around the time of the delivery, as she has been unable to get pregnant since then.

"Do we not have the right to know what our mothers went through?" asks Linda, a member of the Stz'minus (Chemainus) First Nation. She pauses a moment, then expresses a thought in the minds of so many survivors: "What's happening to our bodies?"

Ray Silver, from the Fraser Valley, reminisces about persistent hunger, how he and his brother would sneak away from school to the dump behind a little store near the Grey Bridge to forage for scraps. He recalls asking a friend, "Can I eat your apple core?" Greg from the Gitxsan Nation speaks of having an eardrum broken at age four when he was struck by Arthur Plint—the same staff member who was convicted and sentenced to eleven years for sexual abuse—and requiring a mastoid operation years later. "Eardrops and aspirin were the only medications provided." I can hear the frustration in his voice.

"All this residential school shit doesn't go away."

Julia, also from the Gitxsan Nation, thanks Mosby for giving her people "more voice" and inviting him to speak in her region as well. A Tsartlip member asks why First Nations voices are not being heard and then answers her own question: "No one is listening." Luke George wonders about other kinds of experiments, a question on the minds of many in the audience. It's a subject I've been pondering as well, given the number of stories I've heard about mysterious injections, liquid concoctions, gratuitous surgical experiments. Dr. Dorothy Sam Williams, chief of medical staff at West Coast General Hospital, describes the findings as a "horrific crime that reeks of cruelty and injustice," and suggests that hunger, nutritional experiments, and other residential school experiences were contributors to abnormal

First Nations relationships with food and can be linked to metabolic disorders—hypoglycemia, type 2 diabetes, high blood pressure, and stroke.

One of the most telling observations that comes from Mosby's article is a comment by the officials themselves, who travelled to northern Manitoba communities such as Norway House, God's Lake, and The Pas to assess the suitability of the target population for nutritional experiments:

> It is not unlikely that many characteristics, such as shiftlessness, indolence, improvidence and inertia, so long regarded as inherent or hereditary traits in the Indian race may, at the root, be really the manifestations of malnutrition. Furthermore, it is highly probable that their great susceptibility to many diseases, paramount amongst which is tuberculosis, may be directly attributable to their high degree of malnutrition arising from lack of proper foods.[9]

This statement flies in the face of both prevailing assumptions and medical ethics and gives the lie to those who believe that genetic inferiority made Indigenous people more susceptible to disease. And it raises important questions about the morals of medical experts and bureaucrats who would exploit the sick and starving for so-called scientific purposes, rather than feeding and healing them.

Mosby considers these experiments in the light of the then newly established Nuremberg Code of experimental research ethics:

> During the war and early post-war period, bureaucrats, doctors, and scientists recognized the problems of hunger and malnutrition, yet increasingly came to view Aboriginal bodies as 'experimental materials' and residential schools and Aboriginal communities as kinds of 'laboratories' that they could use to pursue a number of different political and professional interests.[10]

Here his argument concurs with the findings and writings of Mary-Ellen Kelm in *Colonizing Bodies*:

> Aboriginal ill-health was created not just by faceless pathogens but by the colonial policies and practices of the Canadian government. Second, it purports that Euro-Canadian medicine, as

practised among the First Nations, served that colonial agenda, and that its alleged superiority was culturally constructed.[11]

I've been hoping to interview Ian Mosby during his visit to the coast, but he's too busy, surrounded by those who want to talk, welcome him, and honour him for his work. We agree to continue our conversation by email and phone. A few days earlier, I came across an online post he published on *ActiveHistory.ca* entitled, "Of History and Headlines: Reflections of an Accidental Public Historian," in which he discusses the impact of social media in spreading the word. Most importantly, he acknowledges the role played by his privileged position:

> It is, in many ways, a depressing commentary on contemporary Canadian society that such stories were not taken seriously by the government or the media until they were published in an academic journal by a white, male, settler historian. But it is also an important reminder for myself and for other historians that we are often writing from a position of extreme privilege. While academics can use this position to be powerful allies to Indigenous peoples, all too often this privilege is used by settler academics to either speak *for* Indigenous peoples or to advance their careers and interests at the expense of the communities that they're claiming to be experts on.

It's an important reminder to contemplate as I make my way home in a treacherous rainstorm, inches from the edge of the narrow, winding road carved out of the slope skirting the south side of Cameron Lake. Poor night vision does not help. Which will be more difficult to navigate, this highway with its curves and poor visibility or the writing task ahead, given my own blinkered, white perceptions and position of privilege?

68
—

nine

Biological Warfare

O ne of the missing pieces in the long history of Indigenous health in British Columbia, and perhaps the rest of Canada, is the question of smallpox. Where did it come from, how did it spread, and why did it decimate the Indigenous population and not the settler one? The standard answer is that the disease arrived in Victoria on two legs by ship from California, infected the local and northern Indigenous people living in the city, and then made its way into the various parts of the territory by boat and canoe as they fled to their home communities or set off on trading missions to other tribes. As for excessive Indigenous deaths, that was attributed to their reputed lack of immunity to foreign diseases. The lucky settlers, by contrast, had historical immunity and available vaccines. This is a comfortable but flawed explanation for such a great tragedy, perhaps the greatest in Canadian history, and one that allows settlers to feel less troubled about their collective past.

However, over the last 150 years Indigenous people have contradicted the settler narrative, suggesting that smallpox was deliberately and systematically introduced throughout what is now British Columbia to decimate local populations, especially in locations where speculators were itching to take control of Indigenous lands for the purposes of settlement, trade, and resource extraction. What this amounts to, according to oral history, or tribal memory, is ethnic cleansing by means of biological warfare. Scholars, official historians, and politicians have been quick to deny such charges, though some acknowledge the possible small-scale use of infected blankets. Of course, it's their job to consider and evaluate evidence, a practice that has been too quick to ignore oral testimony and too slow to closely scrutinize existing documents. The following comment, apparently made in 1960 and recorded by Suzanne Storie and Jennifer Gould in 1973, appears again in an article by Michael Harkin of the University of Wyoming, a reminder that the threat and origins of smallpox are very present in the minds of Indigenous individuals in British Columbia:

> And the white people get tired of the Indians going over there [Victoria] and they try to chase them away. Well, sometimes they sneak around, and they have some disease with them, this smallpox disease. The Indians see them put something in the bow (of a canoe) and put it, put it way in. So when they are against the wind it blows right to the stern and everybody will catch it.[12]

Debate about the deliberate spread of smallpox is not new. When similar accusations have been made in the US, they were followed by a huge outpouring of dissent and denial, despite very clear intentions in the correspondence between Lord Jeffrey Amherst, commander-in-chief of the occupying British troops in America, and Captain Simeon Ecuyer. Here's Amherst writing to his subordinate: "Could it not be contrived to send the *Small Pox* among those disaffected tribes of Indians? We must on this occasion use every stratagem in our power to reduce them."[13] He suggests that Ecuyer also "try Every other method that can serve to Extirpate this Execrable Race." Ecuyer was more than willing; in fact, he was gung-ho to exterminate the Indigenous people outright: "I would rather chuse the liberty to kill any savage." A clincher in the US case, as if one were necessary, is the written testimony of William Trent, commander of the Pittsburgh local militia: "We gave them two Blankets and a Handkerchief out of the Small Pox Hospital. I hope it will have the desired effect."[14]

In Canada, we have long been in denial that anything so diabolical could have happened here. Biological warfare? Not us. No way. And yet, we've seen, thanks to James Daschuk's *Clearing the Plains* and the work of other writers, how the Indigenous people of the Great Plains were deliberately starved to lessen their numbers and render them incapable of defending their lands, and

70
-

that it was the policy of John A. Macdonald's government to do so. We have also seen how residential schools and the segregated Indian hospitals treated the original inhabitants as if they were a disposable, not-quite-human species, using children as punching bags, sex objects, slave labour, and guinea pigs for drug, surgical, and nutritional experiments. Even today, it's still considered acceptable that thousands of Indigenous people live below the poverty line, their quality of health, education, housing, and social services far below that available to non-Indigenous Canadians. Why is it such a leap, then, to believe that our methods of ethnic cleansing also included the use of smallpox blankets and deliberate exposure to infected individuals?

The publication of *The True Story of Canada's "War" of Extermination on the Pacific*, by writer and lawyer Tom Swanky, has made avoiding that conclusion increasingly difficult. In fact, the provincial government of British Columbia was so convinced of the authenticity of Swanky's claims of deliberate smallpox infection that they publicly exonerated the six Tsilhqot'in chiefs who were hung for murder in the early 1860s. Swanky's book demonstrates that the chiefs had acted in self-defence and that their trials were a judicial mockery. In response to Swanky's research, British Columbia premier Christy Clark offered an official apology in the provincial legislature on October 23, 2014, declaring the chiefs not guilty of the crime of murder and exonerating them fully, on the grounds that, in attacking the settlers who threatened them with more smallpox, they were trying to protect their people from extermination. In short, they had been at war for their own nation's survival. At the end of her speech, Clark also acknowledged the appropriateness of the Tsilhqot'in people regarding these brave but unfortunate forebears as heroes.

Swanky's research suggests that George Cary, attorney general of the colony and legal advisor and confidant of Governor James Douglas, sent a group of men under the direction of Francis Poole through Tsilhqot'in territory on behalf of two companies in which he had shares: the Bentinck Arm Company and the Bute Inlet group called the New Aberdeen Land Syndicate. According to historical documents, Poole admitted dropping off smallpox-infected men in villages along the way, the start of an extermination campaign that would ultimately kill off at least two-thirds of the Tsilhqot'in people and result in even greater ravages elsewhere in the three western colonies. Threats by the settlers to spread the disease further prompted the Tsilhoqt'in chiefs to declare war. Interestingly, the otherwise meticulously kept official records for the colony are intact except for the two-year period in question, 1862 to 1864, when most of the smallpox deaths occurred. These missing documents add considerable weight to Swanky's argument about top-level involvement in the unfolding genocide. Not only does this information contradict the narrative of peaceful settlement, but it also opens doors to future legal challenges and provides grounds for compensation.

The intriguing story of Reverend John Sheepshanks was first brought to my attention two years earlier. Sheepshanks came to BC as chaplain of the Royal Engineers, was a guest of Colonel Moody, travelled extensively in the interior, then returned rather precipitously to England, eventually becoming bishop of Norwich and a member of the House of Lords. In his ghost-written memoir of these times, *A Bishop in the Rough*, published before he died and apparently based on Sheepshank's diaries, the bishop claims to have vaccinated and thereby "saved" all but five of the La Fontaine tribe in the interior. According to Swanky and oral histories, however, this is a lie; in fact, the tribe was so decimated that surviving leader Tsil'husalst had to recruit outsiders to rebuild the La Fontaine ranks.

Swanky speculates that Sheepshanks, who had no medical experience, did not vaccinate them with non-infectious anti-bodies, but deliberately inoculated members of the La Fontaine group with the more virulent live cowpox vaccine, which does not kill the recipient but leaves him extremely infectious for a two-week extended period. The recipient survives, but those in contact with him don't. That may point to a devious truth behind the version of history Sheepshank offers. The trail of deaths appears to have followed him from place to place. It's difficult to believe that also offering the good news of Christ's resurrection provided much consolation to these doomed, infected souls.

72

The blatant racism and high-handedness of the Douglas regime suggests that anything was possible to guarantee the take-over of Indigenous lands, especially if it reduced the chances of outright war, which would have been inevitable at a time when the settlers were greatly outnumbered. Superior technology, in terms of weapons, ships, and vaccines, was not enough to prevent protracted conflict and an inevitable bloodbath. Various tribes had indicated that co-existence was possible, in some cases even mutually beneficial, but they did not support plans that would see them displaced from their villages and traditional territories. Rapid encroachment, bullying, and lack of respect did not sit well with the proud and beleaguered Tsilhqot'in.

Swanky's search for the true story about smallpox matters to me, not only for its rewriting of colonial history by providing a counternarrative, but also because it indicates that our ongoing disregard for the health and wellbeing of BC's First Nations has roots in both the racist policies of the federal government and the colonial administration of James Douglas. The fact that Douglas was married to an Indigenous woman does not seem to have made him more solicitous of the rights and health of original inhabitants in his assumed jurisdiction. Vaccines readily available were not dispensed to vulnerable individuals and nations, and official orders to move susceptible groups from one infected location to another were given in such a way that the likelihood of contracting smallpox greatly increased. Whether he initiated or spearheaded the deliberately induced epidemic, Governor Douglas was certainly cognizant of the plan and the political and economic benefits to be derived therefrom.

The smallpox trail also further explains the long-term suspicion that Indigenous peoples have not only of settler medicine, but also of the motives and integrity of those whose task is to administer it. Equally important, this infectious trail adds weight to the charges of genocide mounting nationwide and that the government works so hard to discourage. Try getting unfettered access to residential school and segregated Indian hospital records and you'll see what I mean. Canada is still in denial, evidenced most recently by the initial refusal of the new Canadian Museum for Human Rights in Winnipeg to use the word genocide to describe Canada's treatment of Indigenous peoples. Response of the Aboriginal People's Television Network (APTN) was swift, quoting Chief Murray Clearsky: "Your museum's decision not to identify the shameful deceit, marginalization and ongoing attempts to assimilate and eradicate the original peoples of this country is a huge slap in the face for First Nations."

The APTN report also draws attention to the efforts of former chief of the Assembly of First Nations Phil Fontaine and Bernie Farber, former executive director of the Canadian Jewish Congress, to have Canada's treatment of Indigenous peoples recognized as genocide on July 19, 2013. Similar reports in other media quote UN rapporteur James Anaya as saying, "It is difficult to reconcile Canada's well-developed legal framework and general prosperity with the human rights problems faced by indigenous peoples in Canada that have reached crisis proportions."

An article from July 19, 2013, in the *Toronto Star*, attributed to Phil Fontaine, along with Dr. Michael Dan and Bernie Farber, president and senior vice-president respectively of Gemini Power Corporation, is titled, "A Canadian Genocide in Search of a Name," and has the following subheading: "Canadians need to face the sad truth that the country engaged in a deliberate policy of attempted genocide against First Nations people." It's hardly surprising, given the neglect and violence inflicted on Joanie's people and other Indigenous populations in Canada, which included deliberate smallpox infection, that subsequent health care has been, at best, a low priority.

Lost Ancestors

A thin gauze of fog hangs over Canoe Pass, a spidery web not exactly obscuring the evergreens on Penelakut Island, but giving them a ghostly aspect, quite in keeping with my limited perspective on Indigenous issues. As I write this I have just returned from a series of cross-Canada interviews with Indigenous Elders, during which I was introduced by phone to Saul Day in Armstrong, Ontario, whose mother died mysteriously at the Brandon Sanatorium.

Doreen Day's roommates at the sanatorium said she looked well before the operation and was ready to go home, but she died on the operating table. Nothing was ever reported about the cause of her death—was it a gratuitous operation, a last-minute sterilization gone wrong? Her burial place is still unknown to the family. This has caused Saul and his relatives a lifetime of grief. He drove to Brandon once to seek information, only to find the sanatorium closed, converted to other use, and no one knew what had happened to its medical records. As I was on my way to Winnipeg, I promised Saul I would make inquiries at the Manitoba Archives.

A couple of hours at the Archives produced no information about the Brandon San, although burial records for the settler population were extensive. Just as I was leaving, the archivist gave me a sheet of paper with a phone number for Manitoba Health, which had a special help-line. I called the number and explained that Doreen Day, who might have been registered under her maiden name of Rae, had died in the early 1950s when Saul was five and already in residential school. Sharon, at the other end of the phone line, offered to search for information. I waited a couple of weeks, then phoned back, but she had come up empty-handed. I could understand the lack of closure Saul felt, having lost my own mother when I was seven and she was thirty-five. I knew her cause of death, but had not been allowed to attend the funeral and had no idea where her ashes were buried, or scattered. As I write, the search for information about Saul's mother continues.

So much residential school and segregated Indian hospital history has to do with lost children whose graves are unknown to their families, the records probably lost or destroyed by the institutions responsible for the burials or by government and religious bureaucracies wanting to cover up the high number of deaths. At a certain point, principals were told by Indian Affairs to stop recording deaths, for the same reason that they shelved Peter Bryce's report on the 40 to 60 per cent death rate in the residential schools in 1907: statistics don't always make for good advertising.[15] Given the importance of burial and paying homage to ancestors in Indigenous cultures, the government's refusal to return the bodies or inform families of the cause of death and place of interment is both an example of crass disrespect and yet another betrayal of trust. Some settler families who have left their ancestors behind in other countries may find this difficult to understand.

Looking back at what has happened here on the coast amongst Joanie's relatives, friends, and Indigenous neighbours and forward to what awaits us in the prairies and central and eastern Canada, it's impossible to overestimate the importance of ancestors and of memory. Here, for example, are the words of Evelyn Voyageur, an Elder-in-Residence at North Island College in Comox, who survived residential school, went on to become a registered nurse, and eventually completed a doctorate. She had a few good things to say about her post-secondary experiences, but admitted, towards the end of her lengthy testimony in Laurie Meijer Drees's *Healing Histories*, that much needs to be known about the impact of the Indian hospitals on the lives and health of First Nations peoples:

Our people that went there were guinea pigs—I'm not sure if you know, but a lot of people today who were in the hospitals, many have only one lung. They did lobectomies on lungs, removed lungs and all those kinds of things. I've heard many stories, even about people who didn't have tuberculosis being put in the Indian hospitals. The hospitals got money from the government for the number of patients they had. The patients were often there for years. And there was a lot of research being done on people. New surgeries and drugs were tried.

These kinds of things were in the back of my mind when I was looking to understand what was happening to our people. Especially when I went to northern Alberta and saw things written in the charts about how people were treated at the Indian hospitals. The Camsell patients were sterilized and there was little consent. I read those things in patient charts. Some of the patients I met were victims of this Indian hospital system. It was quite disturbing for me. Children would die in the Indian hospitals and they were buried wherever. I know examples of where that happened. It was almost like the parents had no say whatsoever in their children's lives once those children were in the hospital. Sometimes parents never even knew where their children were sent. Not much of this seems to be documented.[16]

Considering Evelyn Voyageur's mention of the Charles Camsell Hospital in Edmonton, it is worth noting that this hospital was also the mainstay for Inuit from the western Arctic suffering from tuberculosis, an epidemic that struck at least one out of seven. Their remoteness from the rest of Canada did not spare them from the more virulent European maladies, nor were facilities in the north adequate to treat these diseases, particularly TB. Life in the hospitals or sanatoria had its problems, especially if you did not speak English or French and no one else spoke your language. But the major trauma came from separation. Ships carried off Inuit from the eastern Arctic for treatment in Quebec or at the Mountain Sanatorium in Hamilton, but for those in the western regions, airplanes were the only means of transporting them south to Edmonton. Although wide-scale x-ray detection identified those most at risk, many problems resulted from sloppy bookkeeping. As Inuit often had no surnames, the numbers assigned to them—and worn like military dog-tags—were sometimes lost, making it impossible to inform families in the case of a death and difficult to know where to return survivors after treatment. Given the length of treatment and poorly kept records, many of the survivors never found their way home at all, their fate a mystery to families.

However, the major problem facing Inuit was the brutally abrupt separation from families and communities. As a result of a simple x-ray survey, unlucky victims would be held on board ship or airlifted without explanation. Threat of fog, falling tides, bad weather, or tight schedules resulted in hasty or precipitous departures and separations. The lack of sensitivity during evacuations that might tear an infant from its mother's breast, prohibited people from making proper farewells and survival arrangements for those left behind, and even denied them the opportunity to gather necessary personal belongings. The effect was not unlike being kidnapped or shanghaied, the medical team assuming the role of pirates running a death-ship. As a result many Inuit took to the hills at the first sight, or sound, of the Eastern Arctic Patrol Vessel *C.D. Howe*.

In her instructive treatise, *A Long Way from Home: The Tuberculosis Epidemic Among the Inuit*, Pat Sandiford Grygier comes to the conclusion that the human failings in dealing with this disease—insensitivity, under-funding—amongst our northernmost citizens have their roots in racism:

> Perhaps the main reason was one of which many of the government workers may not even have been aware, because they were so much a part of it, so immersed in it, that it seemed entirely normal; namely, the prevailing colonial, paternalistic attitudes of the period in which they had been reared. Nowadays, such attitudes have become so unacceptable to many people that even mention that they used to exist is sometimes seen as evidence that one has a racist attitude. Revisionist history is not confined to communist societies, nor are prejudice and racism limited to whites. But in the early part of the century, there was generally the smug—and ignorant—assumption among white societies that they were superior

to the local people who lived off the land that the whites coveted; and that, in the case of the Arctic, they were bringing the benefits of civilization to the Inuit.[17]

I'm not convinced that such attitudes are unacceptable today in Canada. My interviews with Elders across the country suggest that racism directed against Indigenous people and immigrants of colour is very much alive. However, I agree with Grygier that too much emphasis was placed on "the purely physical aspects of disease" while ignoring emotions, family, culture, and environment in the healing process.

The trauma of separation from loved ones was only the beginning of the troubles facing Inuit TB patients. Once they arrived in Edmonton or the Mountain Hospital in Hamilton, they lost all connection with family and their place of origin. In the words of Robert Williamson, quoted by Grygier, getting home was not so easy either:

> But in many cases they had been traumatized by their experiences in the south and were apprehensive as to what they might find when they got home . . . [T]hey had no idea . . . who had survived or who had given up on them . . .
>
> And for the younger ones, . . . the hospital and nurses had become home and the only people they knew, and going into the Arctic was going into the unknown . . . Many of them were little southerners, with southern consumption needs and entertainment needs and language usages, with very little in common with the parents who yearned for them back home.[18]

It's fairly clear from reading Grygier's work that logistics was not the main problem in the treatment of Inuit tuberculosis but, once again, systemic racism. She quotes Anglican minister Brian Burrows on the subject:

> They did not think the Eskimo people were worthy of being informed of where they precisely were and didn't think it important that relatives should be informed, that parents should be told where their children were. There was none of that. The authorities didn't think it important that they should get their names right . . .

And the basic thing behind that, I think, is that they refused to believe that they were people.[19]

Robert Williamson concurred: "The humblest and youngest Hudson's Bay clerk may feel that he has authority over the most dignified and respected old Inuk."

The problem was not simply bookkeeping, but the lack of respect for cultural memory. My friend Colin Browne, a celebrated poet and film-maker, has some moving thoughts on these matters to share in an interview with Peter Grant in the *Pacific Rim Review of Books*:

Before literacy, you had to maintain the graves of your ancestors, and, implicitly, their stories, their lineages, their lives. With the development of printing and bookmaking technologies you no longer needed to live near your ancestors' graves; you could travel. You could, in a sense, carry the graves of your ancestors with you. Their memory—their names and stories, their city's and their nation's stories—could be transmitted typographically. Culture—which depends on a profound and continuous relationship with one's ancestors and with one's ancestral territory—became por-table. There is a tribe of us wandering the earth with books under our arms, books filled with the graves of our ancestors. In our journeying we've cut ourselves loose from their graves and the practices associated with them. Many of us have pulled ourselves away from that world.[20]

I found this passage deeply moving as I know how much Colin values his own ancestors, having spent so many years researching, writing, and mak-ing films about them, honouring their passage on the earth. He has no difficulty understanding the value placed on such matters by Indigenous peoples.

While working on a film about the destruction of sacred burial sites on Vancouver Island and the Gulf Islands by real-estate developers, he was in regular contact with the First Nations. As he explains to the interviewer, "I was invited to various locations, and was deeply moved to learn a little bit about what it means to live among one's ancestors; it occurred to me that the majority of the people in the world share their daily lives with their ancestors. It was a humbling thought."[21] His travels took him to the nearby town where I catch the ferry to Thetis and where my neighbours catch the same boat to Penelakut.

"We travelled one day to one of the gravesites," he said, "and as we motored south in a boat from Chemainus my guide pointed to and named every beach and headland along the way. He told me who'd lived there in the not-so-old days, and who was still present. He told me the name of each place, and translated the names for me. He created in my mind a map that has never existed on paper, a vital map of lived lives. This is what I'm trying to do with my poems—to make a map that doesn't yet exist, but is there nevertheless."

These words resonate with me because I consider myself part of the same tribe of writers trying to map lives and territories, doing what Joseph Conrad called rescue work, catching "the vanishing fragments of memory and giving them the permanence of art." I don't know if my mother's ashes were buried or scattered along the stretch of ocean from Fisherman's Cove to Point Atkinson, where she used to swim alongside the boat when she was younger and still in good health. I recall moments together, and I know a few stories about her from the family's albums and collective memory. The rest I imagine and try to reconstruct.

I feel that way about the experiences shared with me by Joanie's people, too, so many of them in precarious health and with so little time remaining, their suffering and triumphs unrecorded, each anecdote a sacred point in time not to be profaned or forgotten.

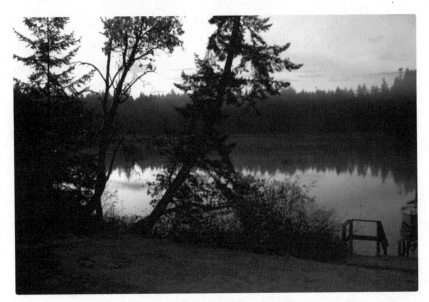

↑ Early morning, looking across at Penelakut (Kuper) Island. **GARY GEDDES**

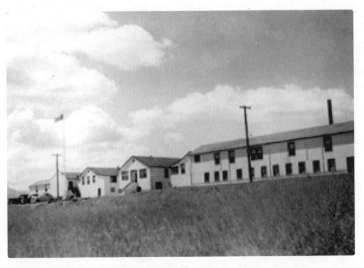

↑ Nanaimo Indian Hospital, circa 1948. **JOAN MORRIS COLLECTION**

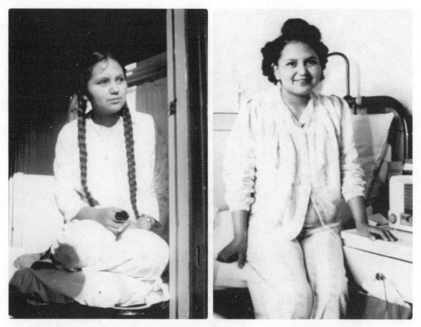

↑ *left*—Mary Theresa Morris, Joan's mother, upon her arrival at Nanaimo Indian Hospital.
right—Mary Theresa Morris, shortly after arriving at Nanaimo Indian Hospital.
JOAN MORRIS COLLECTION

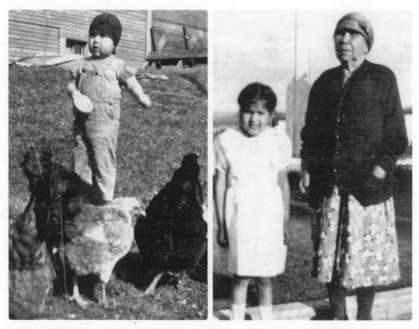

↑ *left*—Joan and friends, Chatham Island. *right*—Joan and her great-grandmother.
JOAN MORRIS COLLECTION

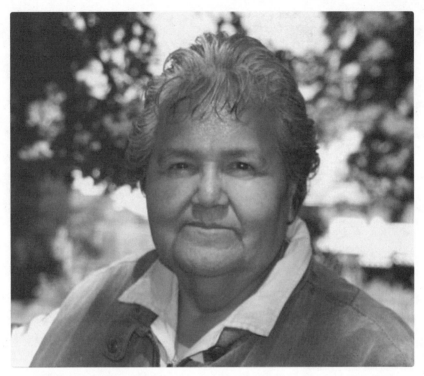

↑ Joan Morris. GARY GEDDES

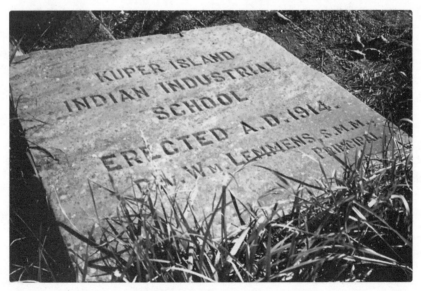

↑ Cornerstone (Kuper Island Indian Residential School). PETER CAMPBELL

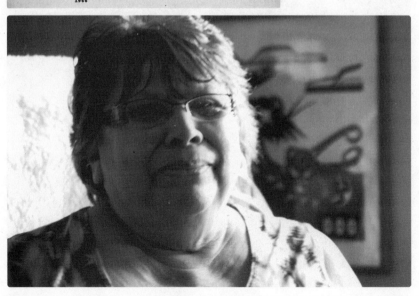

← Richard Thomas death certificate.
PROVINCE OF BRITISH COLUMBIA

↑ Belvie Brebber, at home amongst the Cowichan First Nation, Duncan, BC. **GARY GEDDES**

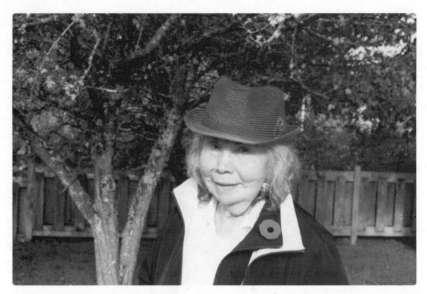

↑ Gloria Nicolson in Victoria. GARY GEDDES

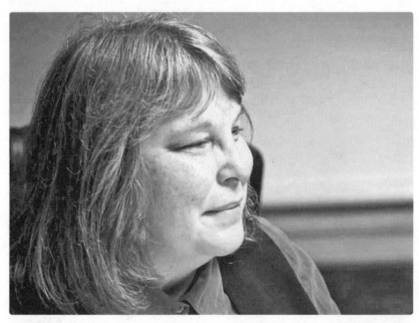

↑ Kim Recalma-Clutesi. PETER CRASS

PART TWO

HEART-LAND

Where the Cure Can Be Worse Than the Disease

eleven

Marilyn, Misery, and Scalps

T estimonies shared by survivors indicate that residential schools and segregated Indian hospitals were often in cahoots, the former serving as farm teams or recruiting grounds for the latter, ensuring full funding and a captive clientele of guinea pigs. It's a harsh indictment that leaves many Canadians aghast. The first stories I heard of this practice involved BC hospitals—the segregated Nanaimo Indian Hospital and the general, church-run R.W. Large Memorial Hospital in Bella Bella. I thought it might be a regional phenomenon related to remote locations and backward politics. But then I heard from four former patients of the Charles Camsell Hospital in Edmonton, whose stories were similar and equally disturbing.

In September 2013, I attended the Truth and Reconciliation Commission hearings in Vancouver. I had brought with me several hundred copies of the brochure I'd had printed that explained my interest in talking with survivors—or knowledgeable families and friends—who'd experienced the segregated Indian hospitals or had difficulties with Canada's health-care system. Marilyn Murray-Allison happened to pick up one of those brochures and opened it to the centrefold image of the Camsell, where she had been a patient as a child. The hospital began its varied career in 1913 as the Jesuit College for Boys. It was taken over by the US Army in 1942, then transformed into a hospital for First Nations, Métis, and Inuit after the war, from 1946 to 1966, one of the largest segregated

89

medical facilities in Western Canada, with superior equipment and better staff than many of the smaller Indian hospitals. But, like similar institutions, it was run on assumptions of Indigenous inferiority and greater susceptibility to disease.

A few days after the hearings, Marilyn sent me an email:

My Mother and I were both patients at that hospital in the early '50s. I was five and a half years of age. We lived in the NWT. My sister Pamela (born in 1949) and I (1946) were born in Yellowknife. My Dad was born in Scotland, my Mother the daughter of an English Hudson Bay man and his wife Maria Vittrekwa, a Gwich'in native from Arctic Red River.

I was in pain and could not sit or stand. Consequently my parents, sister and I were flown to Edmonton to be diagnosed. It was found that I had TB in the lymph gland and my Mother, now deceased, TB in the lung. It was a very tragic time. In a matter of a few hours, our family was separated.

Pamela was taken to our Scottish grandparents' home in Edmonton where she was not really wanted. My Grandmother was terrified when she knew there was TB in the family. My Dad then offered Pam to one of his brothers, Alec, and his wife Thelma and family who already had four children. They accepted her and loved her as long as they could. Times were difficult. The country was still recovering from the war.

Our Mother's TB was contagious, mine was not.

I was separated from all my family and could only occasionally see my little sister several stories up out the window of the Hospital. At three and a half she soon forgot who we were.

All I remember of those days was the hurt and sadness and crying for my Mother and my family. I was dying of heartbreak, not being able to eat and biting my fingernails until they were bleeding. Finally when it was realized that I was not getting better, I was put in a room next to my Mother's, where a wall and a glass window separated us. I was able to see my Mother through the window and began to heal slowly.

Occasionally a kind nurse would wrap my frail body in a blanket and sneak me in to cuddle and see my Mother. By this time (about our 18th month [in the hospital]) my mother was in better health having had one lobe of her lung removed.

*I had been bed-ridden for so long that I had forgotten how to
walk and had to learn all over again.*

*The room was filled with many other Inuit and native children. My
Dad and my Aunts and Uncles brought gifts to me when they could. In
the night the other children, taken from as far as Gjoa Haven in the High
Arctic (not sure why I remember that) in the room would climb out of
their beds and (I think) take my toys and presents and I would not have
them anymore. I remember being given a beautiful little record player
and was not able to enjoy it. It had been taken. I cried a lot.*

Nothing could be a stronger statement of the importance of family and
the folly of separating children from their parents than her comment
about "beginning to heal slowly" when placed in the adjoining room with
a glass partition through which she could see her mother, and the value
of those occasional nurse-assisted cuddles. There are many lessons to be
learned about healing, but one is most surely the role of emotional and
psychological wellbeing in the process of fighting disease. For Marilyn,
unfortunately, the suffering did not end when she was released from the
hospital:

*One day my Dad came to get me. Again I was separated from my Mother,
and I was taken to an elderly couple's home where my sister was staying as well. They were abusive people but they were being paid to care
for us. They were not physically abusive but mentally abusive in many
ways. Pam and I only had each other and were not included as family
unless our Dad was visiting. We ate fried egg sandwiches every day for
lunch. We hid them in our toy box and dreaded the day we were supervised as we "cleaned out" our toy box on Saturdays. To this day we do not
eat fried eggs.*

*We were not allowed to come inside between meals unless invited in.
We were afraid to ask to come in to use the bathroom. You can imagine
how we dealt with that.*

*One day our Dad came to get us and the three of us flew off to
Uranium City, Saskatchewan, to be cared for by my Father's sister, a
woman with a lot of anger, herself having been abused by her husband of
only a few years. Her anger resonated.*

Not long after, my Mother joined us. I will never forget that day, the best day of my life. She was pale and thin but beautiful in her powder blue suit as she arrived at the airport.

In closing, this week has brought back many memories. I also carry the stories in my mind of my Dear Mother's days in the Residential School in Fort Resolution, NWT.

I know some of my story is not related to Canada's Indian hospitals but do hope the little information will help you in your writings.

After reading Marilyn's email, I wanted to know more about her experiences in the hospital and hoped that the TRC hearings and my invitation to talk might restart the process of recall. Also, there were things I wanted to ask her about neglect and abuse in the foster care system, but that would have to wait. Later the same day, Marilyn sent me a postscript describing the terrible health problems that beset her three children:

I had three beautiful children, all three have been afflicted by various diseases at a young age. My eldest son had cancer in the lymph node at the age of 39 . . . my youngest son developed type 1 diabetes at age 25 and my daughter died suddenly in school of "idiopathic pulmonary hypertension" at the age of 13. Her arteries had become so thickened that she had the internal body of an 85-year-old. I have so often wondered why they were all afflicted with diseases such as these.

Why were these things happening? Toxins in the environment? Living upstream from the pulp mill in Kamloops, BC? What startled me as much as those possibilities was a short addition to her email that was typed in all uppercase letters and red font:

I DO NOT REMEMBER DETAILS BUT THERE WAS AN OCCASION WHEN I WAS BLEEDING VAGINALLY AND IT WAS REPORTED THAT I HAD FALLEN OFF OF THE BEDSIDE TABLE THAT I STOOD ON TO LOOK THROUGH THE WINDOW AT MY MOTHER. I DO NOT KNOW WHY THIS STAYS IN MY MIND AND WHY I REMEMBER NOTHING MORE ABOUT IT.

It struck me immediately as problematic, since vaginal bleeding in a child is more likely to be the result of sexual abuse than falling off a bedside table. I did not want to query Marilyn on this subject, but the fact that the story and its improbable explanation were red-flagged indicated that it still troubled her.

When I arrive at Marilyn's home in a lovely secluded subdivision in the View Royal neighbourhood of Victoria a few weeks after our initial correspondence, I see that she has prepared a lunch of soup and sandwiches. In this social atmosphere, our conversation ranges more widely than I'd expected. We speak of racism, and she tells me about visiting her father's relatives in Scotland, who'd hidden all the carving knives in advance of her visit because of stories they'd heard about Indians scalping people. She reminded them that whites had been the first to practice scalping in the Americas. Marilyn is very upbeat, telling me her mother had also been a very positive person who preferred to recall only the good things about her life, hardly mentioning her time in residential school. Marilyn never pressed her on the subject, having escaped that fate herself thanks to her mixed parentage and her non-Indigenous father's connections.

I ask about her children, whom she had written to me about earlier. I knew that her elder son had been diagnosed with cancer of the lymph nodes at age thirty-nine, her younger son had developed type 1 diabetes at age twenty-five, and her daughter had died suddenly at age thirteen of "idiopathic pulmonary hypertension," her arteries severely blocked. I had incorrectly assumed that her sons had both died of their illnesses as well, so I am happy to hear this is not the case, her older son's cancer in remission and the diabetic able to control his illness. Her daughter's death, however, had been a terrible shock. She had been diagnosed early, and although she was slowing down and confining herself more and more to books and a sedentary life, she looked relatively healthy. As Marilyn talks, it is clear that her daughter had known all along her illness was terminal and had not wanted to alarm her parents. Marilyn breaks down while telling the story and begins to weep.

"And all my friends call me the happy one, the life of the party," she says, wiping her tears away with a napkin and managing a sad smile. "That loss ruined my life and my marriage, and made me overprotect my sons and ignore their emotional needs."

Not knowing what to say, I reach out and hold her hand. I can hardly hold back my own tears, the loss of a child being my greatest fear. Marilyn stands up and beckons me to follow her to the back room, where a large photographic portrait of her daughter hangs on the wall, a beautiful teen-ager from whose eyes an unexpected wisdom seemed to emanate.

"I think she's an old soul," I find myself saying, aware of my own doubt about such notions. "She knew a lot more than her age would suggest."

Marilyn nods. "I feel so lucky to have had those thirteen years with her."

I phone Marilyn a few weeks later about returning the copy she'd loaned me of Alice Blondin-Perrin's memoir, *My Heart Shook Like a Drum*. She mentions that she is getting ready to go to Scotland again for a house-sit and plans to visit the relative she'd told me about earlier, the one who hid all the carving knives on Marilyn's first visit. I suggest some sort of revenge, but Marilyn is several steps ahead of me.

"I'm going to buy and gift-wrap a second-hand wig from Value Village, add a few fake bloodstains, and put it under the Christmas tree."

twelve

Linda, Watson Lake, and the Camsell _____

T he first image: a small child in striped pyjamas, three years old, peering through the bars of a crib directly into the lens of the camera. There's intelligence in her eyes, but no indication of pleasure or recognition. Just a quiet, cautious curiosity. She's holding a naked, hairless rubber doll. Behind her, off-kilter on the wall, are two framed drawings, one of a kitten, the other of a girl hugging a rabbit. The scene is a ward in the Charles Camsell Indian Hospital in Edmonton; the year, 1960; the child, Linda McDonald from the Liard First Nation in Yukon, recently diagnosed with tuberculosis. The solitude and vulnerability emanating from the photograph are not surprising, given her age and the abruptness of her departure:

> My earliest memory is of mom walking with me to the little lake we lived beside. She carried me in her arms and she was crying. That is all I remember of mom saying good-bye. I then recall being on a plane with someone.

Her arrival at the Camsell was no less traumatic:

> The bathroom seemed very large. A nurse all in white was taking my clothes off and making me stand in a shower. I think this was my first shower experience. I was crying and she said "shut-up" and banged my head against the wall of the shower. I remember the smell of the bathroom, the large bars of Ivory soap.

Another of Linda's Camsell memories involves being awakened in the middle of the night by a siren, by shouting and people running, and not knowing what was happening. A head-count on the lawn would have revealed someone was missing. As a former Camsell orderly explained years later, hospital policy was to place small children face down at night, their hands tied to the sides of the crib to keep them from jumping up and down. So a nurse must have used scissors to cut the cloth bonds that tied Linda to the crib and carried her out where the rest were gathered.

Linda's email arrived from Watson Lake, Yukon, a few days after my initial correspondence with Marilyn, with the following admission:

> I picked up your brochure at the recent . . . event in Vancouver. I am a member of the Liard First Nation . . . I was in the Charles Camsell Hospital in Edmonton from 1960 to 1962 approximately. I was three years old and returned home just before I turned five. I went in an Indian girl and came out a white girl. It was a very sad time in my life.

As a teacher of Kaska language and culture, Linda proved to be both eloquent and determined to make good use of my interest in her hospital experience.

> I can't wait to be able to talk to you. I have had a life-time of "issues," and one is abandonment. I absolutely know that it started in with my hospital experience.

Over the course of our subsequent correspondence, many emails were exchanged, including Linda's life story, a beautiful, informative piece written at her niece's request. "My Special Childhood" begins at the beginning:

> I was born on a cold December day in 1957, on my family's trap line north of Watson Lake, Yukon. We were a Kaska family, living off the proceeds from trapping and my dad's seasonal work as a labourer and hunting guide. My mom called me a two lynx baby because she was on the trap line the day before I was born, and she caught two lynx. She considered this to be good luck. She was alone checking her traps as was often the case, because at the time dad was working away from home. Her dogs accompanied her, a team of three or four. At home were my six older

siblings who helped out while mom and dad were away. Mom returned in the evening and had me the next morning in her bed like she did with most of her other babies. My older brother John was born on the trail, while mom and dad were hunting moose. Doctor's visits or pre-natal check-ups or tests were non-existent. My family rarely saw a doctor in those days, and one did not seek medical help until you first exhausted your own abilities to heal yourself, or you were on your death bed. Gramma was not at my birth, nor was my aunt, even though they lived not far away. I think it was because mom didn't send my siblings to go for help. Thus mom delivered me without the assistance of another adult. I think my older sisters may have helped by keeping the younger ones out of the way. It's hard to imagine assisting yourself through labour and cutting the umbilical cord of your own baby. That was my mom. She was a strong, self-reliant woman, with a soft heart. My mom could do just about anything my dad could do including making snowshoes. They both shared all the tasks of running a household like ours including shooting and skinning a moose, cutting and hauling wood, snaring wolves (difficult job as they are very cunning) and many other jobs required to simply stay alive.

As this brief account suggests and as the essay further illustrates, Linda's family was mostly independent and self-sufficient, seldom making use of doctors or hospitals. However, one of their saddest moments came as a result of a "professional" misdiagnosis of her youngest sibling:

My younger brother George, who was a year younger than I, died of pneumonia at the age of two. Mom told me the story when I was older, that she brought George to see the doctor in town, but he kept telling her there was nothing wrong with George. Many years later, I met a nurse who worked in Watson Lake and she corroborated mom's story and added that the doctor was a drunk. She said "he was out of it half the time." I don't remember George, but I do remember my Dad holding me as he cried and being treated special.

This story, which is far too common in smaller communities, helps to explain the frustrations and anger Indigenous people in Canada have over their second-rate health care and why Linda and a number of her friends make the long journey from Watson Lake to Whitehorse when they need medical attention.

I decided to check out the record of the Watson Lake Hospital online to see if the situation there had changed in half a century. The town is not exactly remote, situated on the Alaska Highway, yet it seems to have trouble attracting talented and committed medical professionals. At least this is what comes across periodically in the news. A CBC news report from 2013, with the headline, "Watson Lake Families Seek Answers from Yukon Hospital Corp," tells the story of two apparently preventable deaths, one a sixty-year-old named Mary Johnny who died of a bowel obstruction and the other a twenty-year-old named Jamie Porter who was treated for an injured shoulder after a fall on the ice. The temporary doctor sent Porter home, but ordered x-rays the next day, which showed no fractures. He told the patient to take Tylenol and put ice on his shoulder. Porter collapsed a day later and died the same evening. According to the coroner's report, "the progression of what appeared to be such a minor shoulder injury towards sepsis and eventually sudden death of this young man is startling." Even more startling is the fact that this story may be typical of the situation in other communities, some larger than Watson Lake. Porter's uncle, Jim Wolftail, came to the inevitable conclusion: "I shouldn't believe the people at the hospital . . . I should have done more, as a parent. I should have brought him to Whitehorse. You know, why did I wait so long?"

As for Mary Johnny, the coroner's report was even more damning. He blamed the death on a "misdiagnosis" of alcohol withdrawal, a frequent assumption when Indigenous people seek treatment. Both Indigenous families were left asking, "Who will be accountable for these deaths?"[1]

Dara Culhane Speck, in *An Error in Judgement: The Politics of Medical Care in an Indian/White Community*, raises similar questions regarding the inquest and provincial inquiry into the death of eleven-year-old Renee Smith at Alert Bay, insisting that the justice system is stacked against Indigenous medical victims, most of whom are blamed by lawyers and witnesses who trot out all the standard stereotypes. Rather than address the structural problems in the delivery of Indigenous health care, the inquiry's recommendations were to give the hospital an Indian name and hire a local priest to mediate future disputes.[2]

Fifteen months after my initial email correspondence with Linda, my wife and I visit Yukon. Linda is not available when we first arrive at Watson Lake but has arranged to meet us later in Whitehorse. Watson Lake straddles the Alaska Highway, and had once been the staging ground for American construction crews and a pit stop for the intrepid, mostly female, pilots who flew lend-lease aircraft along the Alaska–Siberia route, a dangerous journey over unforgiving wilderness with sub-zero temperatures and unpredictable weather. Of the eight thousand planes sent along this route to help defend the Russian front against Hitler's forces, 174 did not make it.

Ann and I stay at the historic Air Force Lodge, a charming, squeaky-clean log structure, which consists of a central lodge-cum-fuselage with, appropriately, residential wings on either side. We are not exactly high flyers, having camped along the way and arrived by car to do a joint reading, Ann from her new novel, I from a book of selected poems. A few faithful townsfolk gather at the library for the reading, after which Ann and I luxuriate in the good fortune of showers and a comfortable bed instead of sleeping bags on hard ground. We also enjoy some lively conversation with the charming host, a lover of motorcycles and the North and a proud guardian of this piece of history with its delightful memorabilia, including a World War II recruitment poster, a classic Harley-Davidson ad, and a flyer that said, with good post-war diplomacy, "Proudly Canadian" and "*Wir sprechen Deutsch.*"

Segregated hospitals, such as those in Nanaimo and Edmonton, and residential schools all have their origin in the treaties and the Indian Act. Treaty 7, signed between the Crown and First Nations in Southern Alberta in 1877, came with no promise of medical assistance—not even the mention of a medicine chest, as guaranteed in Treaty 6. Treaty 8, which covered Northern Alberta, BC, and part of the NWT, didn't either. A secondary report by Indian Commissioner David Laird promised that "supplies of medicines would be put in the charge of persons selected by the Government at different points, and would be distributed free to those of the Indians who might require them."[3] Laird and his contemporaries assured the Indigenous signatories that "the Government would always be ready to avail itself of any opportunity of affording medical service,"[4] but these promises were not written into the treaty itself. The government subsequently paid little attention to the health of First Nations for several decades.

Although it was preceded by the Blood Hospital, opened in 1893 by the Catholic Grey Nuns, and the much smaller Blackfoot Revival Hospital established by the Anglican Church in the early 1900s, the Camsell was one of the first of the publicly funded segregated Indian hospitals in Alberta. *The Camsell Mosaic*, a book published by the Charles Camsell Hospital's history committee, has many stories about the devotion, hard work, and compassion of the hospital administrators and medical staff. And of course there are letters from patients thanking the doctors and nurses and recounting good experiences. Dr. William Barclay, however, acknowledged the medical limitations under which the staff worked and the measures taken to treat patients "with little or no evidence as to their effectiveness."

When the Camsell first opened, he explains, there were no drugs available for the treatment of tuberculosis.

> Bed rest, surgical collapse of the lung, and fixation of joints by plaster made up our therapeutic armamentarium. We employed these treatments more on blind faith and trust than on any scientific evidence that they were effective. Rest was the cornerstone of therapy and its was rigorously enforced through six routines of activity. Routine "1" was total bed rest and the patient barely moved, even to feed himself. Routines were changed as Meltzer [another doctor] judged the disease to be improving or worsening, and the patients' hopes rose and fell as they either moved up or down the activity scale. With no television, few radios and many of the patients unable to read and hospitalized far away from home and friends, it was a cruel existence.[5]

Barclay's candid portrayal of medical ignorance is followed by a generous tribute to the heroism of a young Inuit boy, Donald Ayalik, who had been severely burned while trying to save his stepfather and young sister after a marine explosion and fire. Hospital staff built a tank from sheet metal in which to immerse Donald up to his neck in a saline solution. Barclay and his wife Margaret, also a doctor, "spent hours placing pinch grafts, from what little skin he had left, onto the burned areas. He developed tendon contractures that had to be surgically corrected and he suffered multiple setbacks from infections. I never met anyone before or since with the courage that he displayed. We will never forget him."[6] After such heroic efforts, the feeling must have been mutual.

In an interview conducted by Laurie Meijer Drees for *Healing Histories: Stories from Canada's Indian Hospitals*, retired nurse Marjorie Warke paints a contrasting picture of the Camsell. Although the hospital was drab, with old iron cribs, and was definitely "not a bright, cheerful place," she remembers camaraderie amongst the nursing staff and a good relationship with patients. She describes a young child who died in her arms and how she often comforted children suffering from separation anxiety. Life in the Indian hospitals was obviously a mixed blessing. Patients were dislocated and separated from family, language, and culture, though lifelong friendships and new skills (reading, writing, music, crafts) were sometimes acquired.[7] Not surprisingly in a book celebrating the hospital and its achievements, the photos show mostly smiling faces of children and adults, busy with projects or posing with friends in wards. However, from what I have learned thus far, it's impossible not to wonder how many of those photos were staged and how many smiles forced.

As a counter to my growing cynicism about the segregated system, I hear in Whitehorse a mostly positive account of the Camsell from Linda's friend Roger Ellis. I've been trying to reach Roger for several days; he's already missed one appointment due to mechanical problems with his truck. When I finally meet him and his wife Tina, I see he's replaced the truck with a shiny late-model SUV painted candy-apple red with silver flecks embedded in the base colour. After introducing ourselves, Roger, Tina, and I stand on the sidewalk for a few minutes checking out the new purchase and admiring the paint job.

Whitehorse has changed a lot in the past twenty years. The gravel roads have been paved, and many new building sadded, including large box stores. The upscale Kwanlin Dun Cultural Centre and the attached branch of the Yukon Public Library both command priority locations along the banks of the Yukon River, transforming the city from a frontier town composed mostly of bars to a modern northern metropolis. But the restaurant we have agreed on for lunch, which has come recommended by friends, is a welcome exception to the trend.

Klondike Rib and Salmon on 2nd Avenue claims to operate in the oldest building in town. Originally a bakery tent, it morphed phoenix-like into a freight depot, post office, coffin factory, and finally its present incarnation as a local hotspot diner constructed of timber and corrugated iron with an unobstructed view of hills across the Yukon River valley. As we settle into lunch at the rough-hewn tables covered with pink-and-white checkered oilcloths, Roger describes his experience at the Camsell. He'd been struck twice by lightning in his teens in Yukon and was transported by plane to Edmonton, where the large team of doctors gathered around his bed pronounced his case hopeless. His systems had closed down and the poisons were spreading throughout his body. He rallied enough to sit up and protest the diagnosis.

"Shit, you guys are supposed to be experts. Get me someone who knows what he's doing." With that, and a few added expletives for emphasis, he collapsed back on the bed. Shortly after, Dr. Edward Romanowski took on the case and stuck several long needles into Roger's body to drain off the poisons.

"The fluids started pouring out of me. I resembled a colander. Years later, I went back to the Camsell to thank Doctor Romanowski, but the receptionist brushed me off because I was an Indian, saying the doctor was on his rounds and could not be disturbed. I pestered her and insisted that she mention me by name. She finally gave in, made the call, and suddenly started addressing me as 'Sir.' Moments later, Dr. Romanowski stepped out of the elevator, burst into tears and gave me a huge hug."

During our meeting in Whitehorse and in subsequent phone conversations, Linda has never expressed her feelings about the segregated hospital system and its impact on Indigenous people more strongly than in this email that came a few weeks later:

> So many First Nations people shifted from relying on their own knowledge and power and put so much faith in Western Medicine. People didn't

stand up for themselves, like my mother who knew her baby was very ill. She was helpless to say anything to defy the doctor or resist in any way. People had so little power. So many stories, even today, of people who are ill because of some misunderstanding or something they missed in the system, re: helping people. I was talking to a woman in Watson Lake, two days ago. She came to visit me, a young 51-year-old woman, who has been healthy pretty much her whole life, but she has breast cancer and it went undetected, because she did not understand the system of booking a mammogram, so she let it go by for years. She was also treated rudely by a few doctors she saw, re: "a feeling that something was wrong with her breast." Now she has breast cancer and luckily it has not metastasized but she is very upset. I hear stories all the time, of people not knowing what to do, where to go or how to deal with some ailment. Often it starts out small and then it's a huge problem later on, because they didn't understand or put off doing something, because they didn't want to have to deal with the hospital or doctors. People avoid doctors and the hospital at all costs.

As I'm learning, bit by bit, the Camsell story is not just about the failures or successes of a specific hospital, but about larger systemic problems created by a belief in the superiority of Western medical knowledge, a dismissal of traditional practices, and racist assumptions that have left some Indigenous peoples in hell, and many others in limbo.

thirteen

Melinda, Medicine, and John A. _____

Among the many Camsell photos in *Healing Histories* and in the federal government's archives, one touched me deeply. It shows eleven children, aged two or three, in white gowns arranged on benches by a nurse wearing a face mask. The two toddlers in the front row wear moccasins, another is missing a shoe, and a third sucks her fingers. Collectively, the photograph does not depict a single mood, such as fear or anguish or pleasure, though the little ones are anything but animated. However, I know how children need the love and affection of parents, and how their health can plummet and immune systems give up without this special care, and the photo sends a shiver down my spine. I know, too, that many of those toddlers, if they made it through their hospital ordeal, were not sent home but shipped off immediately to residential schools, where their chance of survival was sometimes as low as 50 per cent.

Relevant to the history of Indian hospitals are Canada's long-standing policies of ignoring Indigenous wellbeing and deliberately starving First Nations populations to make them more easily manipulated and subservient to the demands of white settlement. Many of the great chiefs, including Poundmaker and Big Bear, were brought to their knees as beggars, asking for handouts to save their people. As Maureen Lux explains in *Medicine That Walks: Disease, Medicine and Canadian Plains Native People, 1880–1940*, the violence that erupted at Frog Lake and elsewhere was precipitated by hunger. "The starvation at Fort Walsh," she observed, "was a cynical and deliberate plan to press the government's advantage and force the Cree from the area and allow the government a free hand in developing the prairie."[8]

It has taken more than one hundred years to dismantle some of the myths about Canada's Indigenous peoples, including the notion that they are more susceptible to disease than other populations. Hunger, malnutrition, overcrowding on tiny reserves, and captivity in residential schools that were havens for sadists and paedophiles—none of this was particularly good for the immune system. Continual abuse caused fatalities that might have been avoided, or at least been less widespread, in earlier times when buffalo and game were plentiful and when confidence and solidarity were not in short supply. These trials, which I believe amounted to genocide in slow motion, were approved at the highest level of government. Prime Minister John A. Macdonald made this evident in 1882 when he assured the House, "We cannot allow them to die for want of food," but added that Indian Commissioner Edgar Dewdney and the Indian agents "are doing all they can, by refusing food until the Indians are on the verge of starvation, to reduce the expense."[9]

The Department of Indian Affairs was no less complicit in the neglect of Indigenous health in Alberta and other jurisdictions. After Dr. Peter Bryce, chief medical officer of the Department of Immigration, was sent out to study the conditions in prairie residential schools in 1907, he wrote a serious and disturbing report about the overcrowding, malnutrition, and alarming death rate in the schools (estimated at 40 to 60 per cent) that he had witnessed. At the time of his appointment as chief medical officer, Bryce was considered eminently qualified for the task by his superiors. However, after he reported that 24 per cent of the residential school students died during the first fifteen years of the operation of the schools, with the notable exception of the File Hills Residential School in Saskatchewan, which reported a 75 per cent death rate over a similar period, his popularity plummeted. Even after he'd been sidelined by Indian Affairs, Bryce pointed out that his strategy with vaccines and isolation of the worst cases among new immigrants had been successful, saving lives and reducing the spread of tuberculosis, and would work well with the Indigenous population, he continued to be ignored and dismissed as "troublesome."

That conditions were appalling and deadly in the thirty-five schools Bryce visited in Alberta, Saskatchewan, and Manitoba is borne out by the statistics he provides. Duncan Campbell Scott's refusal to act on this information confirms that the government had no intention of reducing the death rate from tuberculosis amongst the Indigenous population.

In his eventual publication, *The Story of a National Crime: Being an Appeal for Justice to the Indians of Canada; the Wards of the Nation, Our Allies in the Revolutionary War, Our Brothers-in-arms in the Great War,* Bryce acknowledges not only the long-term contributions of Indigenous peoples, but also the government's responsibility for their medical care. This text, published in 1922 and sold for 32 cents, is advertised as a "Record of the Health Conditions of the Indians of Canada from 1904 to 1921." After being ignored, vilified, and forcefully retired from government service, Bryce spared no effort to lay the blame for those thousands of cruel and unnecessary deaths on D.C. Scott and the federal government for their parsimony, inertia, and "criminal disregard for the treaty pledges." What's notably missing from this list of accusations is the word *racism*, which seems to have been the root cause of such neglect: disrespect for Indigenous peoples, the prevailing belief amongst the government and general settler population that they are inferior and of less value.

On April 12, 1910, three years after Bryce's original findings were shelved and the position he held was eventually eliminated, Scott conceded the overall accuracy of his former employee's claims, but dismissed the need for action: "It is readily acknowledged that Indian children lose their natural resistance to illness by habitating so closely in these schools, and that they die at a much higher rate than in their villages. But this alone does not justify a change in the policy of this Department, which is geared towards the final solution of our Indian Problem."[10]

Somewhat later, Scott would add, "It is only necessary to carry out some common sense reforms to remove the imputation that the Department is careless of the interests of the children."[11] As the NFB film *Duncan Campbell Scott: The Poet and the Indians* implies, the fact that Scott's own daughter Elizabeth died of scarlet fever in a European boarding school in 1906 at age eleven is a clear indication that his blindness on the perils of removing children from their families was not confined to the workplace.

The promised reforms, of course, did not come. Maureen Lux tells us that Chief Long Lodge, whose people had been forcibly removed from Fort Walsh and were sick from starvation, put the matter bluntly: "I want no government medicine. What I want is medicine that walks. Send three oxen to be killed and give fresh meat to my people and they will get better."[12] When the Indigenous people—devastated, drastically reduced in numbers—refused to disappear, residential schools and Indian hospitals were the next phase of the "final solution" that Indian Affairs had set in motion.

Laurie Meijer Drees makes a case for the Camsell Hospital as a more enlightened and caring institution than most, the responsibility having passed from religious institutions to government, where one might hope, despite the foregoing evidence to the contrary, bodies could be given as much attention as souls. Eventually, in terms of medical procedure, less emphasis was placed on confinement and absolute immobility for TB patients. Still, the continued existence of segregated hospitals was a clear indication that systemic racism was alive and well in Canada.

Forced sterilization, confirmed by several Indigenous Elders, including retired nurse Evelyn Voyageur, along with gratuitous drug and surgical experiments, continued to happen at the Camsell and in many Indian hospitals. Teeth were often removed without freezing. Drugs were administered that caused discomfort or worse; deaths were falsely reported to authorities and families often not informed. Sexual abuse was not uncommon, as countless testimonies at the hearings of the Truth and Reconciliation Commission confirm. Much of the fear that First Nations, Métis, and Inuit have of doctors and hospitals today derives from the unpleasant experiences and racist attitudes in these institutions.

Something Lux has to say about the Camsell in *Medicine That Walks* reminds me of Joan Morris's story of her uncle Ivan barely escaping death at the surgeon's hands in the Nanaimo Indian Hospital. Lux quotes a Blood Elder as saying that the Camsell was known as the place patients were sent to from which "they never came back." She links this perception to "the number of thoracoplasties performed there. In this procedure, a lung was collapsed permanently and ribs were removed. Major surgery created its own dangers, and removal of the ribs resulted in significant blood loss and high mortality. Survivors were badly disfigured; some were given wax prostheses to keep their chests from collapsing altogether."[13] How ironic, given these primitive medical procedures, which resemble crude resource extraction practices, that the Charles Camsell Hospital was named after the Deputy Minister of Mines and Resources.

As I try to weigh the pros and cons—the service of dedicated medical practitioners and the cynical decisions of government—in addressing the issues of Indigenous health in Alberta, the phone rings.

"I saw one of your brochures at the TRC in Vancouver," the voice on the other end says. "I was in the hospital in Edmonton from age four and a half to eight and a half. Yes, the Charles Camsell—and it ruined my life. My great-great grandfather visited me once, but was not allowed to come again. I saw a lot of things, every kind of abuse. I remember the casts, little kids with hips and both legs in a body cast, just a small hole where they could pee. At night, the orderlies would be doing things in those holes."

A strong voice, urgent and articulate, proceeds to tell me about how her knees were small for her size from being bed-ridden for so long at the Camsell, but she still became an athlete. She was one of eleven siblings from the Blood Reserve in Alberta, twenty kilometres from the US–Canada border.

"After the Camsell, I had one month at home before being sent to residential school, St. Paul's Anglican. I left the reserve without enough time to get acquainted with my sisters. After four years I didn't remember what they looked like. And we'd been in the same school, too."

Eventually, Melinda Bullshields offers her name. She is calling from Vancouver where she rents a tiny flat on 2nd Avenue near Commercial Drive, two blocks from where I spent part of my own dysfunctional, impoverished childhood.

"They groomed me for solitude," Melinda explains. "I coped with the abuse by dissociation, closing off the emotions, being elsewhere when nasty things happened to me."

This situation continued back home on the reserve, where Melinda's sisters tormented her for being too English and where the worst abuses learned in residential school and Indian hospitals had become an epidemic. When we meet later, at a coffee shop on The Drive, Melinda shows me her copy of *The Camsell Mosaic* and turns to the photo of herself on page 211, front row, third from the left, one of ten tiny, costumed girls, part of the Counterpane Players, wearing a frilly, conical cap. It's her only photo of herself from that period, a possibly lighter moment, though one she does not remember, in an otherwise dark period.

"I hate both sides," she says, "so where does that leave me?"

And where does this confusing and disturbing legacy leave us? It's definitely an invitation to rethink attitudes. All Indian hospital records that have not been destroyed should be made available immediately. And the years spent in Indian hospitals, as a result of deliberate or unwitting exposure to tuberculosis in the residential schools, should be considered in the financial compensation process. A symbolic gesture to jump-start the reconciliation process might be to begin with the Charles Camsell Indian Hospital.

After twenty years of serving as an Indian hospital, the Camsell was converted into a hospital for the entire population in 1967. The general hospital remained open until 1996, when it closed, in part, because of asbestos contamination. There was talk of renovating and turning it into housing for Edmonton's homeless and low-income population, a large number of whom are Indigenous. As a result of community protests, it was decided, instead, to sell the building to developers, who promised to turn it into condos for seniors and yuppies. It remained abandoned for years, grew increasingly decrepit, and only made the news when it periodically caught fire or was mentioned as part of the Internet ghost-watch. Hearing that the asbestos has been removed from the building, I contacted the Edmonton City Council and suggested that it would represent a major and welcome attitudinal shift if they were to purchase the structure and proceed with an earlier proposal to turn it into low-income housing.

In *Unsettling the Settler Within*, Paulette Regan suggests we stop talking about the Indian problem and start talking about the settler problem, the racism and the greed for land and resources that keep First Nations people, not, as their new designation suggests, at the head table where decisions are made, but somewhere in the lobby, cap-in-hand, or toiling in the scullery. One thing's certain: apologies are not enough. Harold Cardinal wrote many years ago in *The Unjust Society* that equality of health or education services is not enough: "We aren't starting on equal grounds. Equality of services doesn't mean a thing to people who are so far behind they can't even see the starting line. It just means we would remain that far behind. That's not good enough. We want to catch up. Then we can talk equality."[14] Cardinal, who was born in High Prairie, Alberta, and grew up on the Sucker Creek Cree Reserve, wrote those words in 1969. Some forty-seven years later, we still have not taken them to heart.

I'm in Edmonton's north end now, visiting the site of the Camsell, a forlorn but imposing concrete structure that had once been a red-brick edifice surrounded by a firetrap of wooden out-buildings and connective walkways. I can't look at the Camsell shell without sensing the history—not exactly a halo—that surrounds it. From there I drive north to St. Albert, site of the former Edmonton Indian Residential School, where ninety-eight Indigenous patients who did not survive the Camsell, including thirteen babies, are buried on the grounds of the former school. Their names are inscribed on marble slabs on four sides of a monument made of round stones set in concrete. Below the list an engraved inukshuk seems to point to a hovering cross in the sky, intercepted by a feather, perhaps representing the soul of a deceased. On the top of the six-foot-high structure, nestled between the stones, mourners have placed plastic toys and a pink skipping rope with white plastic handles. The cold wind has blown a tiny black plastic car onto the paved surface. I pick it up and replace it on top of the monument, wondering about those who'd left it here, about the decades they've spent suffering the loss of a child.

George Muldoe, a Gitxsan elder from Kispiox, was a student at the Edmonton Indian Residential School from 1951 to 1962. He remembers being assigned on several occasions to burial detail for the nameless Camsell dead delivered to the school to be interred, some in boxes, some wrapped in blankets, some in pieces. He and his pals hacked away for hours, digging graves in the frozen ground. He claims the current site gives a false impression and that the graves were spread around the school grounds haphazardly, so the list of names is not only inaccurate but also incomplete.

Before departing, I drive a few hundred yards farther to Poundmaker's Lodge, a drug and alcohol addiction centre that now occupies the grounds of the former residential school. A stand of poplars in the distance is festooned with long, brightly coloured cloths. I ask a woman outside the centre having a smoke what they signify.

"They're prayer flags," she says. "When the wind blows, they flutter and the pain is carried off by the breeze."

fourteen

Eugenics—Extermination by Another Name_____

Although the Charles Camsell Hospital was less than stellar in the history of Indigenous health care in Western Canada, there were other ethical and Indigenous health issues of equal concern in the province, including Alberta's Eugenics Act of 1928, imitated by British Columbia in 1933. The Act, however well-intentioned—and promoted by otherwise respected and progressive figures such as Tommy Douglas and Nellie McClung—was wrong-headed, based on the false assumption that mental challenges, problematic behaviour patterns, and disabilities were genetic and therefore inheritable.

As we know from the Holocaust, Pol Pot's killing fields in Cambodia, and residential schools here in Canada, governments often dress their hellish activities in good intentions. It's now common knowledge that 300,000 Indigenous women were sterilized in Peru under the leadership of president Alberto Fujimori, supported by USAID, and that the Czechs, from 1973 to 2001, carried out a ruthless sterilization program to reduce the numbers of Roma. Consider the truly chilling Article #5 of the Sexual Sterilization Act:

> If upon examination, the board is unanimously of the opinion that the patient might safely be discharged if the danger of procreation with its attendant risk of multiplication of the evil by transmission to progeny were eliminated, the board may direct in writing such

surgical operation for sexual sterilization of the inmate as may be specified in the written direction and shall appoint some competent surgeon to perform the operation.[15]

What leaps out is "multiplication of the evil," a phrase as telling and perverse as George W. Bush's "axis of evil" to describe those who were at war with American foreign policy and empire building under the banner of globalization. Although the word "evil" was removed from the Act in 1937, to describe physical disabilities or mental illness as evil sounds, to the modern ear, more than slightly medieval. And yet we know that such policies in Canada and the US were admired and copied by the Nazis during World War II and used at the Nuremberg trials to justify medical experiments and exterminations during the Holocaust. While sterilization was often justified as a way to purify the gene pool by eliminating the proliferation of defective genes, there were other less apparent and equally insidious reasons for promoting sterilization: reducing the costs of care for the disabled, socially dysfunctional, criminal, or mentally deficient, obviously a factor in the minds of economists and bureaucrats in charge of the public purse. So, too, was the gradual elimination of certain troubling elements in society, including what Thomas King has pegged as the problematic or "Inconvenient" Indian.

The eugenics acts in Alberta and BC targeted First Nations along with the poor, immigrants, homosexuals, criminals, alcoholics, prostitutes, the disabled, and the feeble-minded. As Indigenous peoples who were "expected to vanish" were somehow surviving years of abuse, disease, starvation, and the genocidal intent of the residential schools, here was another means of "exterminating the brutes," to use the deadly advice uttered by Mr. Kurtz in Conrad's *Heart of Darkness*. In other words, *Indianness*, that category created by the colonizers, could now be viewed as an evil, a disease to be eradicated. It has been estimated that, although First Nations, Métis, and Inuit people represented only 2.3 per cent of the population in Canada in the 1930s, 25 per cent of those sterilized in Alberta were Indigenous people. Given the number of hospital records altered or destroyed, that percentage is likely much higher.

And it's not over. As I write, an email comes from Yvonne Boyer, a Métis author, lawyer, and holder of the Canada Research Chair in

Indigenous Health and Wellbeing at Brandon University, with a link to an article by Betty Ann Adam in the *Saskatoon Star Phoenix* newspaper, dated November 17, 2015. Yvonne comments, "I can't believe forced sterilization is still happening."

The article focuses on the story of Brenda Pelletier who, at age thirty-four, was bullied into agreeing to have her fallopian tubes clamped, on the understanding that the procedure could be reversed. At the last minute, on the operating table, she changed her mind but was ignored because the hospital had a signed permission form. After the operation, the smell of burning flesh made her realize that her tubes had been fused, not clamped. There would be no reversal. In making her story public, she hoped to prevent this kind of coercion from happening to other Indigenous women.

Betty Ann Adam's article and the attached readers' comments are instructive. Pelletier's old friend Tracy Banab had found herself in a similar situation during a Caesarian section delivery, but was fortunate that her obstetrician arrived in time to prevent the sterilization. Two of the commenters admit to having gone through the same involuntary procedure and the distress it caused. While public comments range from sympathetic to harshly judicial, the article focuses mainly on the larger issue of freedom of choice, quoting Karen Stote's important study, *An Act of Genocide: Colonization and the Sterilization of Aboriginal Women*:

> These were not about eugenics per se, but were also about how to most efficiently intervene in what were considered social or public health problems . . . The ideology that justified historical coerced sterilization continues to shape state and medical interventions in the reproductive lives of women, (especially) marginalized, racialized and Indigenous women, pressuring them to get sterilized for their own good, to save them and society from having to care for additional children.[16]

Stote describes the process of sterilization and birth control, promoted among Indigenous peoples, as the "colonization of childbirth," a phrase that leads her, a few pages later in the book, to quote Harold Cardinal's assessment of Canada's Indigenous policy as "a thinly disguised programme of extermination." And Yvonne Boyer, also interviewed on the subject, had

114

this to say: "This has the underpinning of the 'guardian and ward' theory, in which health system staff assume, 'We know what's best for you because we don't believe you're capable of making those decisions on your own.'" She attributes this attitude to the historical fact that Indigenous women have long been "on the bottom rung of the social ladder and because of the other laws and legislation that were targeted against them."[17]

After a century of ignored complaints and petitions from First Nations people, serious pressure on the government to address injustices in the administration of the Indian Act began to build in 1969 when Harold Cardinal published *The Unjust Society*. He wasted no time pussy-footing around troubling issues, including the federal government's intractability:

> Positive steps by the government to fulfil its treaty obligations represent one aspiration common to all Indians. It was for this reason that our people were encouraged by Prime Minister [Pierre] Trudeau's call for the creation of a Just Society. This brief, dazzling flare of hope, however, quickly fizzled out when Mr. Trudeau publicly announced that the federal government was not prepared to guarantee aboriginal rights and that the Canadian government considered the Indian treaties an anomaly not to be tolerated in the Just Society.[18]

Harold Cardinal's dream was to open the eyes of the Canadian public to the shameful conditions in which Indigenous people were living and the racism they faced daily. Stated bluntly, "There is little knowledge of native circumstances in Canada and even less interest. To the native one fact is apparent—the average Canadian does not give a damn." Of the notion that Canada is free from racial prejudice, he is equally blunt: "Statements of this nature are just so much uninformed nonsense."[19]

So, too, the "gross ineptitude" of the Department of Indian Affairs comes in for a serious drubbing:

> To ensure the complete disorganization of native peoples, Indian leadership over the past years and yet today has been discredited and destroyed. Where this was not possible, the bureaucrats have maintained the upper hand by subjecting durable native leaders to endless

exercises in futility, to repeated, pointless reorganizations, to endless barrages of verbal diarrhoea promising never-coming changes.[20]

Cardinal makes the point that politicians and bureaucrats have broadcast the message that Indigenous people are helpess incompetents for so long that they have come to believe their own fictions. Shut up and listen is his advice to the settlers and their government, something they don't want but need to hear. The politics of assimilation and divide-and-conquer must be discontinued. The difficulty lies, he says, in ongoing racism; and this is relevant today, almost fifty years later, as evidenced in the high rates of incarceration among Indigenous people and the deaths and disappearances of Indigenous women and girls.

In a chapter called "The Great Swindle," Cardinal discusses the issue of what was promised in Treaty 8, which I've already mentioned, including the unfulfilled and broken promises of Commissioner David Laird on the subject of medicines. These promised supplies and services, none of them written into the treaty, were minimal at best and often never materialized. Cardinal's conclusion is harsh but justified:

> The truth of the matter is that Canadian Indians simply got swindled. Our forefathers got taken by slick-talking, fork-tongued cheats. It wasn't their fault. Our forefathers, with possibly a few cynical exceptions, never understood the white man. They had fought battles, known victory and defeat, but treachery was new to them. They were accustomed to trusting another man's word, even an enemy's.[21]

Cardinal goes to considerable length to expose government rationales for ignoring, amending, and possibly abolishing the Indian Act. What this amounts to, he insists, is that the Indigenous person can only "earn his place in the Just Society by disappearing." Like the Québécois of thirty years ago, many of whom felt themselves invisible within Canada, Indigenous peoples could not count on the wider public to protect their rights.

> A man who believes Canadian society will grant equality to the Indian because of its sense of Christian responsibility or its adherence to Christian beliefs or because of its obeisance to any

concept of human rights common to all men, believes in myths. The Canadian society, self-righteously proclaiming itself just and civilized, has not extended equality to the Indian over the past century, and there is no reason to believe, expect or hope that it will change its spots over the next century if the Indian stays weak.[22]

Fortunately, Harold Cardinal's call to arms has helped spur into action two generations of powerful men and women, a number of whom I would soon meet in Edmonton.

fifteen

Phantoms, Extinction, and Hunger _____

One of my favourite pieces of art is an etching, a gift from Margaret Nachshen, a well-known and gifted Montreal visual artist and former student at Concordia University. It shows a series of five horses and riders, clearly Indigenous hunters from the Great Plains, emerging from the shadows, each rider carrying a beribboned spear. There's something insubstantial and haunting about these figures, the rider bringing up the rear barely etched in, his mount evidenced only by a pair of seemingly superfluous legs. I think the effect is heightened by the degree of light showing through the bodies of horses and men, as though they are tending towards negative space, and by the unusual shading techniques: tiny starbursts and minute scratches that resemble hairs.

The chest and left arm of the figure in the right foreground are etched into what appear to be layers, depicting either musculature or veins, perhaps both, the left leg disappearing at the edges, the right arm that holds the reins altering from the tiled muscles of the shoulder and upper arm to an intricate web of nerves at the wrist. The right leg has the effect of overlapping folds of muscle or cloth. Taken together, these elements present a rider in perilous shape, a bandaged casualty of war. The central rider sits erect, serious, the outline of his body a sort of palimpsest of markings that resemble the rectangular grid of settlement or the fracture lines of a damaged sculpture.

I think what struck me first about this work was that it seemed to depict a vanishing act, a version of the once popular notion of a people or peoples doomed to disappear, somewhat reminiscent of the ghostly presences in John Newlove's poem "The Pride." The dark, expressionless faces suggested not the walking but the riding dead. Years later, when I began this study, I looked up Margaret Nachshen on the Internet and discovered that the etching is called *Les Cavaliers Fantômes*. I had not connected it with the French-language television series by the same title or with the popular country western song "Ghost Riders in the Sky," which I used to belt out at age ten while hoeing potatoes on the farm in eastern Saskatchewan, the lyrics of which would always make the hair stand up on the back of my neck.

Now that I know and have been entrusted with the testimonies of so many vibrant and successful Indigenous people, and realize—despite phenomenal obstacles in their way—that they are not disappearing, but are the fastest-growing demographic in Canada, Margaret Nachshen's etching has taken on a new meaning for me, not the misplaced nostalgia for a vanishing people but a sense of what could be in store for all of us if the contract between Indigenous and non-Indigenous peoples remains broken. Stan Jones's mournful lyrics, despite their hokey and quasi-religious diction, drift back to me across the years: "As the riders loped on by him he heard one call his name / 'If you wanna save your soul from hell a-ridin on our range / Then cowboy change your ways today or with us you will ride / Tryin to catch the devil's herd across these endless skies.'"

While I don't subscribe to the notion of souls, I am becoming accustomed to the Indigenous respect for and faith in living Elders and those who've passed to "the other side." So I am encouraged to discover the work of non-Indigenous writers who value not only their own heritage, but also that of the original peoples of their adopted land. I'm thinking of Mel Dagg's, *The Women on the Bridge*, a moving fictional reconstruction of the Frog Lake Massacre that makes excellent use of the published accounts of survivors. Another is Candace Savage, who has written a memoir-travelogue-detective story devoted to reconstructing the history of Cypress Hills in southwest Saskatchewan that includes dinosaur bone-beds and a fascinating saga of Indigenous occupation, a people who, unlike the dinosaurs, have somehow managed to resist extinction. It's called *A Geography of Blood* and is as poetic as it is deep. Curiosity brings Candace and her husband to the tiny town of Eastend, and an automotive breakdown keeps them in this place where they eventually uncover displacements and slaughters they had not imagined. She is so taken with the area that she applies for an author's residency at the childhood home of Wallace Stegner, author of the famous prairie novel *Wolf Willow*.

Reading her account, I can't help recalling my own brief prairie childhood outside Yorkton, Saskatchewan, slopping pigs with their muddy pink snouts, being covered in dust from stoking sheaves of wheat, working the cream separator, and being affectionately nicknamed the Saltshaker Kid because of my inability to milk cows. I never mastered the skill of squeezing those dangling, sausage-like teats in a way that would produce more than a few drizzles of white gold, even the waiting cat appalled by my incompetence. And then there were the winter excursions to and from school by horse and toboggan, blowing snow spiced with the periodic whiff of equine farts— muted gunshots punctuating the swish of runners and the horse's rhythmic grunts of exertion. There is no shortage of metaphor in this landscape, if you have the mind and the taste for it, and Savage's prose is kept afloat by its linguistic buoyancy, whether a sky "quilted with clouds" or "the icy bite" of wind. Although she and Keith were sufficiently hooked on the Cypress Hills to purchase a small bungalow within a block of the Stegner house, she did not make her peace with the author of *Wolf Willow*, whose depressingly brutal childhood coloured his view of the prairies and its history.

While the local guidebook provides useful information and recommendations for outings in the Cypress Hills, it does not deliver the whole story. And strangely, to Savage, neither does Stegner's novel. She finds it rich, exhilarating, and layered in meaning—a counter-narrative to the myth of progress that drives much western settlement literature and is still the choice trope of politicians and the Chamber of Commerce—but also disturbingly racist. While Stegner admits that the treatment of Indigenous people in Canada and the US is proof that the Nazis did not invent genocide, Savage takes him to task for his racist comments, including a description of the tribes gathered in the Cypress Hills for sustenance and protection in the 1870s and 1880s as "an ethnic junk heap."[23]

As she spends more time in the Cypress Hills, Savage too becomes a reader of signs: stone circles marking the place of tipis; ceremonial encampments— perhaps that of the great Lakota chief Crazy Horse, later murdered in captivity by the US Army for his part in the defeat of Custer at Little Big Horn—the fading rumble of buffalo, grizzly, and elk driven toward extinction; the massacre of the Nakoda by white wolfers; and bodies of the nameless dead who once peopled this now sparsely populated land. There was money to be made from the slaughter of buffalo, but recorded history uncovers a different agenda. As Savage reminds us, "Colonel Dodge himself once cheerfully announced, 'Every dead buffalo is an Indian gone.'"[24]

With the buffalo wiped out, absolute dependence was guaranteed. Eventually Savage, who describes herself as an "accidental pilgrim" to the Cypress Hills, becomes part of the story, the terrible web of treachery and pain that preceded and followed the treaties. She discards the erroneous notion of an empty land and the imported US myth of Adam and Eve in the New Eden, replacing it with a story of criminal displacement and betrayal, but also, according to her new Blackfoot friend Narcisse, hope. What seemed a silent, almost pastoral land emptied of people turns out to be a storied land, with so much to teach. After taking her on a tour of the sacred sites in southern Saskatchewan and Alberta, Narcisse responds to her inquiries about the possibility of Indigenous cultural recovery: "'Anyway, you newcomers aren't going anywhere, and we aren't going anywhere either. I think it's a viewpoint now of we're in this together.'"[25]

Rescuing the vanishing fragments from the past is a worthy ambition and one that seems to me to be prominent in the minds of many Indigenous and non-Indigenous writers and visual artists, including the poet John Newlove, who was born in Saskatchewan. His writing rings truer each day as we endeavour to understand our troubled history: "the knowledge of / our origins, and where / we are in truth, / whose land this is / and is to be." Two of his best poems, "The Pride" and "Crazy Riel," focus on the wilful extermination of Indigenous peoples. After calling up images of the Pawnee and Sioux, destroyed by white racism and greed, Newlove begins a roll-call of the ghosts of Raven, d'Sonoqua, and the great Indigenous leaders of the Plains: "they are all ready / to be found, the legends / and the people, or / all their ghosts and memories, / whatever is strong enough / to be remembered." In these "roots / and rooted words," Newlove struggles to write "the pride, the grand poem / of our land, of the earth itself."[26]

sixteen

Monkey Business

C lifford Cardinal was ten when his father enrolled him in the special Roman Catholic Day School on Goodfish Lake reserve, two hours northeast of Edmonton. It was a fall day, the round coin-like leaves of the poplars beginning to turn silver, an ambivalent currency for kids as it heralded the end of summer. For their Cree parents, however, many of whom were Catholic converts, the incentives were clear: extra food rations—mainly tinned pork—and the chance for their children to avoid going to the nearby Blue Quills Indian Residential School. The kids would not only get an education, but could also return home every evening, presumably safe from the abuses many of their parents and grandparents had suffered in the compulsory, government-funded and church-run institutions. It seemed like a good deal, but for the cohort of thirty-eight enrolled students it would prove costly, a Faustian bargain that they would pay for with their wellbeing and, finally, their lives.

"We were taught nothing," Clifford recalls, as we drive from Edmonton to Goodfish Lake reserve in his new white pickup, his wife Delores in the backseat checking messages on her cell phone.

"That's not quite true," he says, correcting himself in a low, deep voice, the words taking their time to emerge. "I remember learning the alphabet song and singing it over far too often. The rest of the time we watched television and received a lot of vaccinations. Every three months."

The school, he tells me, which operated for only four years, from 1959 to 1963, was run by a German immigrant named Herman Haënsell and a nurse called Miss Rohlhoff, who administered the oral and injected vaccines.

We left Edmonton around noon, stopping to fuel ourselves and the truck at a gas station with a Tim Horton's, then proceeded through several small towns in the direction of Smokey Lake, where Delores has a scheduled medical appointment. An hour later, Clifford and I stretch out on the hospital lawn to wait.

"Haënsell was a lousy teacher," he tells me, "but very popular with the men in the community who piled into his room to watch *Gunsmoke* on Saturdays and wrestling on Sundays. Some claimed Miss Rohlhoff was trained as a doctor, though she refused to deliver babies."

When Delores joins us again, we do a quick pit stop to give the white pickup a wash it doesn't need and that won't last on the dirt roads. Delores is cautiously optimistic about the Ethiopian doctor from Spruce Grove doing a locum at the hospital.

"Too bad she won't stay long."

On highway 36 north, we turn off on a dirt road to drive twelve kilometres east to the reserve at Goodfish Lake, which Clifford tells me is now called Whitefish Lake First Nation, #128. He's not sure why the name was changed. It's a soft, rolling terrain of small hills and valleys with occasional farms, liveable and inviting. There's no town, no store, just a couple of converging roads and a school that doubles as a community centre. Clifford shows me the site of the infamous RC Day School, which was apparently dismantled and moved. Then we stop briefly at the abandoned nursing station, doors and windows missing, old files and records soaked and rotting in complete disarray on the main floor and in the basement.

We're looking for anything related to the former day school. Clifford dusts off a map that includes the family farm he's inherited just outside the reserve boundaries and sets it aside. I rummage through several piles of mouldy documents scattered amongst broken drawers and bits of plywood cabinet. One folder has a cover whose large print announces in bold white letters against a green background: CHILD WELFARE IN PROGRESS. Below the heading, ironic under the circumstances, are the words: NATIVE CHILD WELFARE SERVICES, PRACTICE GUIDELINES. Nearby, a 1987 report called Indian Oil & Gas Task Force, addressed to "the chiefs," catches my

123

attention, but the ink has smudged on the waterlogged paper. We realize there's only the faintest possibility of finding important documents relating to the school in this mess, and the stench of mould and rot is on the verge of making us sick.

Having dropped Delores off at her sister's place, Clifford takes me to the cemetery where so many of his friends, relatives, and former classmates from the "special" RC Day School are buried. What those children learned is a painful truth: the white man's medicine is not to be trusted. I stop beside Esther's resting place amidst the tall grass, the white paint having disappeared from the edges of the wooden cross. Someone has wrapped a narrow beaded strip, long since faded, around the vertical board, and placed a recent bouquet of pink and white flowers in a plastic container that bears only her first name. Clifford directs me to an elaborate grave, its message etched in granite, with marble urns full of white roses on either side: In Loving Memory, R. Dennis Cardinal, 1954 to 1982. A relative, twenty-eight when he died, a graduate of the special day school, which he had entered at age five.

As we pause beside the tiny clapboard Catholic church that stands watch over the dead, Clifford tells me this is the spot where he saw the priest raping his sister.

"No one would believe me," he recalls. "The priest told people I was disturbed and not to be trusted. I was only ten at the time. I didn't know what he was doing to her then, but I knew it was wrong."

We walk back to the truck, which by now has a fresh coating of dust, and stop in to say hello to a neighbour, introduced as Gloria, whom Clifford has not seen for years. She's out in the backyard working on her flower garden and recognizes him immediately. After introductions and an explanation of what we're doing, she says, "Sure I remember that day school. I was there briefly. It was red." This surprises Clifford, as he does not associate the building with a specific colour.

I'm here because of a thesis Clifford submitted to the University of Alberta in 2000, in which he suggests a link between those vaccines and the high rate of morbidity and mortality amongst his classmates. He refers in his thesis to an *Atlantic Monthly* article by Debbie Bookchin and James Schumacher called "The Virus and the Vaccine," which would lead them to a book-length study with the same title, offering pretty strong evidence that the Salk and Sabin vaccines were contaminated with a cancer-causing simian virus known as SV40. The Salk vaccine was cultivated in a medium composed of the minced kidneys of rhesus monkeys, more than 170,000 of which had been sacrificed in the interests of science, or profit. The formaldehyde solution, known as formalin, was supposed to kill or deactivate the polio virus, and any contaminating viruses present in the minced kidneys. This did not happen; SV40 survived.

So far, we have no new information about the RC Day School, except that it might have been painted red. The questions remain: Who authorized this school? What were they hoping to learn by exposing young kids to excessive doses of two contaminated polio vaccines? And why would anyone do this to children? Such questions occur to me daily while gathering information about First Nations health, in particular those who attended the segregated hospitals. The answer to the final question is obvious: as in the case of the nutritional experiments, they do this to the young, the helpless, and the marginalized because they can, and because it can be done with impunity.

I've sent inquiries and Freedom of Information requests to numerous institutions, including Indigenous and Northern Affairs in Ottawa, Library and Archives Canada, the University of Alberta, and the Catholic diocese in St. Paul. I'm cynical but never without hope that something incriminating but undetected by government lawyers and bureaucrats will show up. However, I know many researchers are finding that the documents they request have been destroyed or had the sensitive material blacked out. We're free, it seems, to examine documents that won't make the government look even worse, or add to the likelihood of litigation and further compensation. Withholding or destroying information vital to the health and wellbeing of the country may be common practice in dictatorships, but it should not be tolerated in what purports to be a democracy.

125

The polio vaccines administered to each child in the Goodfish Lake laboratory-cum-day-school were several times the recommended dosage for polio prevention. The injected Salk or the oral Sabin vaccine were already being widely distributed throughout the United States, Canada, England, and Australia. Both vaccines required only one dose, plus a booster the following year. No one had ever recommended taking both at once, especially over an extended period. What makes this experimental situation even more disturbing is the knowledge that both vaccines were contaminated with SV40, the monkey culture considered an ideal medium in which the polio cells could proliferate. Jonas Salk, whose vaccine hit the market first, thought the formalin (formaldhyde) solution the vaccine was immersed in would kill or deactivate all foreign viruses. However, as early as 1954, Bernice Eddy, suspecting that viruses caused cancer, injected 154 hamsters with cells from rhesus monkey kidneys. To her amazement, 109 of the hamsters developed brain tumours and died. Albert Sabin, who hoped to capitalize on the doubts being cast on the product of his chief competitor, switched to using the kidneys of the green monkey, which he considered to be so clean that his vaccine could be taken live, without the formalin immersion.

Unfortunately for the thirty-eight Cree students at the Goodfish Lake school and, presumably, for the rest of us, Salk and Sabin were both mistaken. The immersion period of Salk's vaccine in formaldehyde was not long enough to kill the SV40 virus. And that same virus, which had mysteriously found its way into the kidneys of the green monkey, showed up in the Sabin oral vaccine as well, probably even more virulent in its natural, or live, state. Evidence of the contamination and its danger to humans was denied, disputed, and kept under wraps for as long as possible, especially by government and the pharmaceutical companies. Too much was at stake in terms of reputation and profit to admit that, thanks to the efforts to eliminate one dreadful disease, another even more virulent pathogen had been released into the human population. SV40 is widely accepted to be a deadly carcinogen and is now considered the most highly researched virus in the world. It's the subject of a book and countless articles; and there's even a website devoted to the issue called SV40 Cancer Foundation. Statistics suggest that SV40 is linked to significant increases of cancer in humans since the 1950s.[27]

How does SV40 function? It knocks out or interferes with the body's natural cancer suppressors. Normal cell reproduction is monitored and controlled by what are called suppressor genes, often compared in scientific articles to the breaking system in a car. The RB1 gene, for example, is the tumour suppressor that is known to impede the replication of an oncogene called the retinoblastoma protein. When RB1 is interfered with so it cannot perform its usual function, the brakes fail and the oncogene proliferates, which gives you the runaway-car condition we call cancer.

A fascinating and disturbing characteristic of the SV40 virus is that it can remain dormant for long periods, like an expert sleeper cell, waiting for just the right conditions to launch an attack. We don't know when it might go into action, debilitating our natural healing capacities, but doubtless this would happen when the body's immune system is at its lowest ebb. The science around SV40 suggested tightening safety regulations or demanding recall of the vaccines, but neither happened.

How do I know any of this, and how did my study of the segregated Indian hospitals lead me to a laboratory disguised as an elementary school on a remote northern Alberta reserve? To answer that question, I need to tell you more about Clifford Cardinal.

Planning to participate in the Edmonton Poetry Festival in April 2015, I made some advance contacts to see if I could arrange interviews with Elders who had experienced the segregated hospitals and sanatoria. One of my contacts proved especially useful, introducing me by email to an amazing woman named Nancy Gibson. Nancy wrote back immediately to say that my project and literary background resonated with her on several levels: first, because of her research as a medical anthropologist in Canada and Sierra Leone; second, because of her decade of working with the Tlicho people in the Northwest Territories, facilitating community health initiatives; and finally, because she was trying to write "a difficult piece about being a white mother who has raised an adopted Métis son, exploring the overlap of the personal and the political in our family for 45 years."

What riveted my attention in her open and generous letter was the following paragraph:

> One of my first graduate students when I began my 10-year career at the U. of Alberta was Clifford Cardinal. He came to me, guided by an elder, to explore the deaths from cancer of many of his classmates. He had recovered from cancer himself, though most of the others had died.

He believed it was from testing in the residential [sic] school they were in,
where no teaching took place, as it was run by a doctor and a nurse. I have
attached his thesis. He is a professor now in the School of Public Health.

I immediately read the attached thesis and was startled by the statistics Clifford Cardinal had provided. Of the cohort of thirty-eight students, in what was not a residential school but a special Roman Catholic Day School on Goodfish Lake reserve in northern Alberta, thirty-one had died by the year 2000, when the thesis was submitted, twenty-five from a variety of cancers, four from car accidents, and two from suicides. The seven remaining survivors, including Clifford, also had encounters with cancer. He had survived the removal of a malignant brain tumour in 1997, which set him on this path of inquiry, but, as I would soon learn, he'd had another malignant brain tumour removed a decade later. By the time Clifford and I met in June 2015, only he and one other Goodfish classmate—she was too riddled with cancer to talk to me—were still alive. In a comparable group of students from the local Protestant day school at Goodfish Lake by the year 2000, where there had been no laboratory testing, there had been seventeen deaths, only seven from cancer.

Clifford speculates in his thesis, not unreasonably, that the high rates of morbidity and mortality amongst his classmates were the result of the testing that had been done in the special day school, where each student received excessive doses of two different polio vaccines: one injection and four oral doses via sugar cube each year from 1959 to 1963.

The SV40 saga is a shocking and gripping account of good intentions, genius, and ambition overwhelmed by greed, deceit, and denial on the part of individuals, industry, and government. In addition to the rivalry between Jonas Salk and Albert Sabin to produce the best vaccine, there were the investments of the pharmaceutical companies and the reputation of government officials in the National Institutes of Health's (NIH) Division of Biological Standards to consider. In the words of Bookchin and Schumacher, authors of *The Virus and the Vaccine*, "In one of the biggest blunders in medical history, nearly half the American population—about one hundred million people—and millions more in Canada and Europe, were administered this widely contaminated vaccine."[28] When Bernice

Eddy's research proved in 1954 that SV40 was a carcinogen, causing brain tumours in hamsters and in all likelihood in humans, every effort was made to discredit Eddy's research, destroy her career, and suppress any information that might cause panic, litigation, and a discrediting of the national vaccination program.

When the incidence of polio cases actually increased rather than decreased following the introduction of the vaccines, authorities not only refused to acknowledge that the dangerous SV40 simian virus had not been deactivated or killed during production, but also failed to increase safety standards. In spite of the growing scandal and *Time* magazine boldly announcing, "There is no doubt, however, that a large part of the Salk vaccine and of the live-virus Sabin vaccines that were used in clinical trials throughout the world were contaminated with SV40 virus,"[29] the US, Canada, Britain, and Australia did not refuse the contaminated stocks. And Big Pharma did not destroy or recall them. This should not surprise anyone, since there is clear evidence, confirmed by television media and the *New York Times*, that Bayer, with FDA approval, deliberately sold abroad HIV-infected Factor 8, a drug for hemophiliacs, causing thousands of deaths, when it had already been pulled from US markets. No one was convicted in the US for this travesty, although some officials in the recipient countries faced prison terms.

By the time Clifford Cardinal's special day school closed down in 1963 and the two-room structure was dismantled, alarm bells were already ringing about the increased incidence of cancer in Australian children. As the evidence mounted against SV40, which Bookchin and Schumacher so brilliantly document, so too did the nasty conspiracy of silence to refute or suppress the facts. Fifty-three years later, with SV40 showing up in cancer tumours in infants and children who never received the contaminated virus (which will be explained in the next chapter) and legal cases against the pharmaceuticals declaring it a deadly substance, officials of the US government's CDC and NIH are still in denial.

In one of those serendipitous moments that researchers long for, my friend Mira Leslie, visiting from Seattle, who trained as a vet and is an expert on infectious diseases in animals, listened to my spiel about SV40 and raised a few objections to Clifford's hypothesis, in particular the question of why there would be further testing of the effects of high doses of Salk and Sabin vaccines when these vaccines had already been used with some success in trials around the world. All I could think to say at the time was that if SV40 were reputed to be a minor cancer risk in then-current doses, how much of an increase in exposure would it take for the contaminating simian virus to constitute a more immediate and dramatic health risk? That's when Mira surprised me by confiding that she was a childhood friend of Debbie Bookchin, a co-author of *The Virus and the Vaccine*, and would put me in touch with this expert on the subject.

seventeen

SV40 and Mother Theresa_____

A s my trip to Library and Archives Canada had proven a waste of
time in terms of gathering relevant information about the rogue RC
Day School at Goodfish Lake, I am very pleased to connect with Debbie
Bookchin. Her book *The Virus and the Vaccine*, co-authored with her husband James Schumacher, is the most comprehensive and compelling
account of the development of the Salk and Sabin polio vaccinations and
the controversy surrounding them. I'd sent her my health brochure and
a draft of my chapter on Clifford Cardinal and his thesis, which she had
shared with her husband and co-author Jim, who was also willing to talk
with me from upstate New York, where he was doing research.

Although not aware of similar tests done elsewhere in Canada or in
the US, Bookchin is not the least surprised by the suggestion that there
were rogue experiments going on. In fact, she has recently read a two-part
article by Marcia Angell in the *New York Review of Books* called "Medical
Research: The Dangers to the Human Subject," a review of a book called
The Ethics Police. The review included a photo of Indigenous children from
St. Ann's Residential School in Ontario, one of the six residential schools
where nutritional experiments had taken place.[30]

Bookchin begins our phone conversation by reminding me that cancer is a multifactorial disease, so it's important to know exactly what kind
of cancers appeared in the cohort of thirty-eight students if a clear link
to SV40 is to be established. The most common brain cancers showing

SV40 are choroid plexus tumours and ependymomas, a link that goes all the way back to Bernice Eddy's hamster research in 1954. Another likely hangout for SV40 sleeper cells is mesothelioma, a cancer that forms in the outer lining of the lungs and has most often been associated with exposure to asbestos. In combination with asbestos, or a similar rock dust found in certain regions of Turkey, SV40 has the best chance of overwhelming our natural immunizing T-cells and contributing to mesothelioma.

I say "contributing" because, as Bookchin's husband and co-author James Schumacher reminds me, even though the bulk of medical researchers agree that SV40 contamination is now widespread, if not universally present, in humans, no one has been able to prove definitively that it causes cancer in our species. Schumacher also recommends that I get exact details about standard doses for the two polio vaccines and compare them to the doses used at Goodfish Lake RC Day School, information that he assumes is available in the literature or from the archives of Connaught Laboratories.

My discussions with these two investigative journalists sends me back to *The Virus and the Vaccine*, which devotes many pages to the renewed research into SV40 that took place in the late 1980s and early 1990s. The combined research of Michele Carbone, Daniel Bergsagel, Robert Garcea, Harvey Pass, Janet Butel, Joseph Melnyk, and John Lednicky into SV40 and the controversy surrounding its use makes it possible for Bookchin and Schumacher to say that the new research provided "incontrovertible proof that the simian virus that had been presumed dead when present in the polio vaccine was alive and kicking, possibly causing cancer decades later in humans."[31] The shocking conclusion that follows is that "the positive brain tumour samples all came from children too young to have received contaminated Salk vaccines. That meant that either SV40 now was being transmitted within the human population or vaccine supplies since 1964 had still been contaminated at the time."[32]

The frequency of SV40 showing up in brain and lung tumours now extended to osteosarcoma, cancer of the long bones, another of the SV40 targets suggested decades earlier. By 1999, researcher Janet Butel could say with confidence, "I'm convinced that SV40 is able to cause infections in children."[33] According to Bookchin and Schumacher, "SV40 had broken out from the original group of Salk vaccines and was apparently here to stay." And the indefatigable Carbone would confide to his interviewers that SV40 is not only one of "the most potent human carcinogens that we know," but also "the smallest perfect war machine ever," a guerrilla cell able to outwit, outwait, and outmanoeuvre our natural tumour suppressors such as the p53 gene.[34]

How does all this play out in the Goodfish Lake case? Considering official restrictions and the blacking out of sensitive documents pertaining to the health and wellbeing of Indigenous peoples, the only other route towards confirmation would be to find uncensored documentation about the approval and running of the school or have all or most of the tumours of members of the cohort who died of cancer tested for SV40 contamination. The likelihood that tumour samples exist or could be located for all the cancer mortalities amongst the Goodfish Lake cohort is small; and coordinating permissions and laboratory tests using polymerase chain reaction (PCR) techniques would be financially prohibitive. Then there is Schumacher's conundrum: even if you find SV40 genes present in significant numbers, how do you prove they caused the cancers?

In my view, the primary source of verification at this late stage lies in the testimony of band member we'll call Miss X and in the boxes Clifford Cardinal believes are stored in her basement, files related to her and her aunt's involvement in the administration of the RC Day School's vaccines. I share these thoughts by email with Clifford, who is caught up in mid-term responsibilities at the University of Alberta's Family Health Services. I'm concerned to let him know that these difficulties in no way question the authenticity of his claims. He's a complicated man who has managed to clear a path that allows him to be a healer and teacher in both the Indigenous and non-Indigenous worlds. In the former, he is very much in demand; in the latter, he is respected by those colleagues who take the time to get to know him and observe his success with students. And, of course, there are those petty racists in the faculty who dismiss or pay no attention to him or take some small pleasure in addressing him as "chief."

We've talked at length about his work as a healer, his brief time as a spiritual adviser for the San Francisco Padres, and his negative experience with the Independent Assessment Process, during which one church

and one government lawyer interviewed him about his brief but tumultuous months at Blue Quills Residential School, where he ran away three
times after witnessing a friend being raped. His compensation package
of $110,000 was withheld, ostensibly because his attendance could not be
verified but also, he feels, because he refused to dismiss his thesis about
Goodfish Lake RC Day School as a fiction. It's a sore point with Clifford,
both the refusal and the effort made to discredit his academic achievements and reputation.

During our brief travels together, Clifford spoke about his work in the
Family Health section at the University of Alberta, where he is a professor and counsellor, and about long-term community relations in Goodfish
Lake, rendered complicated by rivalries between Catholics and Protestants.
The books I've read and the records I've consulted at Library and Archives
Canada provide numerous instances of Indigenous children getting sick
and dying as Christian denominations engaged in heated jurisdictional
battles over their souls, and while federal and provincial departments
argued over who would pay the medical bills. Parents at Goodfish Lake
decided that a single, non-denominational school, well-equipped, would
best serve the interests of the community, but their efforts were thwarted by
the school's nuns, the priest, and the bishop, who cited government regulations regarding the right to religious education. Around the same time,
there were complaints, even among the faithful, about the behaviour and
ethics of Catholic clergy within the community. Clifford's father, responding to such allegations, spearheaded a temporary removal of the priest and
nuns from Goodfish Lake reserve.

As it happened, Mother Theresa, in the years before she became
famous for her work amongst the poor and the dying in Calcutta, was visiting the diocese of St. Paul around the time of the expulsion. She was
recruited for her empathy and diplomatic skills to try to resolve the problems at Goodfish Lake, the aim being to re-establish relations between the
church and the community. According to Clifford, she was quite effective
in that role and much loved by those who met her. During her time on the
reserve, she stayed in the Cardinal household, sharing a bed with nine-
year-old Clifford. When he told me this, on the road back to Edmonton, I
couldn't resist the obvious conclusion.

"You may be the only man who can claim to have slept with Mother Theresa."

Clifford laughed so hard the truck swerved into the loose gravel and required some quick adjustments to stay on the road, a warning from on high that you don't make light of such important matters.

eighteen

Hormones and Healing ————————————————

A nother of the benefits of my time spent in Edmonton was meeting Métis entrepreneur and cultural guru Gary Bosgoed, who has been involved as an adviser and contractor on many Indigenous projects, including the All Nations' Healing Hospital in Fort Qu'Appelle, Saskatchewan. He's a big man, well over six feet tall, but also big-hearted, someone who believes in paying it forward, and he was quick to offer assistance after hearing of my project. When I told him I was heading to Saskatchewan, he said he'd arrange for me to meet some of his friends in Regina and at the Fort Qu'Appelle hospital. Rather than just give me the names and contact information, he flew to Regina, took in a Roughriders game with his son, and met me afterwards at Starbucks in Regina's Southland Mall.

Among the names he recommended that day was Noel Starblanket who, at age twenty-four, became chief of the Starblanket Cree Nation and at twenty-nine grand chief of the National Indian Brotherhood, precursor of the Assembly of First Nations. When Noel and I meet the next day at the University of Regina, where he's an Elder and counsellor, I ask him how he feels about the rebellious younger version of himself in Donald Brittain's 1973 documentary film. Forty-two years later, he's in his late sixties, but has lost none of his confidence or smarts. He smiles affectionately at the character portrayed in that film and dismisses it as part of the arrogance or piss-and-vinegar of youth. Besides, he tells me, there's a more recent film version called *Starblanket: A Spirit Journey,* about the path he has been on in recent years, after recovering from his anger and alcoholism and returning to the teachings of the Elders.

Noel tells me he was chairman of the board of the old Fort Qu'Appelle Indian Hospital while it was administered by the tribal council. The federal government divested its responsibility for Indian Health Services to the provinces in the '50s and '60s, so the provinces began to train Indigenous advisors in the '70s. Old obligations and jurisdictions shifted, though not all of the old attitudes, including the notion that Indigenous health did not merit equal funding. The only abuses Noel recalls were monetary and political ones.

"In downloading to the provinces," he tells me, "they cut back several millions of dollars. The Fort Qu'Appelle Indian Hospital was old, part of it sinking into the ground. Add that to the rising costs of maintaining a building and trying to handle the administrations. The white administrators were only interested in massaging their own credentials: look what we've done to help the Indians. Nice people, but I've been around the block a bit, so I knew what their real concerns were. It came to the point where we almost lost our accreditation. I'll never forget those people who worked so long and hard to help us preserve that accreditation status. I'll take some credit for that. I learned a lot about administration from that work. I was born in that hospital, and my mother died in that hospital."

While he does not have any specific abuses to share, Noel is fully aware of the low status of health care for his people and recalls the frequency with which his father, a chief, used his own truck to bring bodies back from the tuberculosis sanatorium at Fort San to be buried on the reserve. The Métis orderlies would know more, he adds, but they were instructed to keep quiet. "I came in at the moment of devolution, the handing over of the fiduciary responsibilities. Those are the things I know about."

I ask Noel about racism in general, and he is not short of information and opinions.

"The colonial, racist society on which all these institutions were predicated are all based on the same mentality. I spend a lot of time talking about these things in schools, in particular two books written by long-time friends: *American Holocaust,* by David Stannard, and James Daschuk's *Clearing the Plains.* I talk about these books to teachers in training here when we discuss the treaties and the genocide imposed on Indigenous peoples. Cutting out the genitals of native women, such things as imposing disease over sustained periods of time, over hundreds of years. That whole mentality, the remnants remain, in how our federal and provincial governments handle the needs of Indian people. It was a mentality that spoke of us as inferior people."

I mention the racist incidents shared with me by Joanie Morris and Belvie Brebber and my talk the previous day with Larry Oakes, in one of the Indigenous clinics in downtown Regina, who said, "The only thing that will outlast colonialism is racism." Noel recalls a few of his own telling encounters with Euro-Canadian medicine.

"I've had those kinds of experiences too. I'm a diabetic. My doctor here treated me for some thirty years. He didn't have a narrow view of medicine. For example, if I tell him I want to go to a ceremony and take some natural medicines for my diabetes, he believes he should be able to sign off on a requisition allowing this, so I can be reimbursed. When he moved his practice from Fort Qu'Appelle to Regina. I followed him. Anyway, he recommended me to this institution at the Regina General called MEDEC, Metabolic & Diabetes Education Centre. So, I went there. I spoke to a nutritionist, a diabetes nurse, and a doctor. They were all very nice.

"'Well, if it's all the same to you,' I said, 'my doctor has me on about five different kinds of pills, some of which have negative effects on my body. I'd like to drop all but one and supplement it with my own First Nations traditional medicines.' So, they gave me a blast. They said that stuff doesn't work. It's all just a bunch of superstition. And on and on they went. You just follow our rules and our guidelines and you can even defeat diabetes.

"I said, 'Okay, I understand your scientific view, but the body is also connected to the spirit. That's what we believe. We use spirituality in our treatment.'

"They said, 'Well, you have a choice there, you can either continue to be registered with us or not be; it's your choice.'

"'Fine,' I said, 'just keep me registered, if it assuages your conscience, but I'll not be back here.'"

When the talk turns to Indigenous medicines and healing practices, he tells me he's since had a heart attack and another episode of diabetic neuropathy during which one eye ceased to function.

"When my left eye closed, I was sent to a neurologist at the General, who then directed me to an ophthalmologist. He said, 'I'm going to have to do an operation on your eye. I'll get back to you with a date. In the meantime, come back in six weeks and we'll see how it's progressing.'

"So I went to several ceremonies and a healer there said, 'By the end of the ceremony, your eye will begin to open.' And it did. So I went back to the opthalmologist.

"He looked at my eye and said, 'What do you need me for?'

"He sent me back to the neurologist who checked me over and said, 'Whatever you're doing, keep on doing it.' So that was that. And that's a true story."

When I mention Cowichan herbalist Della Rice, whom we've invited twice to Thetis to teach us about medicinal plants, Noel raises the issue of belief, insisting that you really have to believe it's going to help you.

"My experience is that First Nations doctors can't cure everything. They are specialists too. For example, when I had my heart attack, I went to five different places before I found someone who could help me. The cardiologist took another angiogram and found that my vessels had healed. He couldn't understand it. There's credibility, power, and there's proof. As I said, I've been doing this now for thirty-five years. Previous to that, I grew up with it with my grandparents. Then I went to residential school and I went into politics and was away from it for a long time. I discovered it again in 1980."

So Noel has mellowed. That's why he laughs when I point out his youthful speculation in the 1973 film that it might take five or ten more years to sort out the problems between Indigenous and non-Indigenous peoples.

"It isn't over, right?"

"You know, with the acknowledgement of all the abuses heaped upon First Nations, there's a genuine hope for that kind of reconciliation between residential school survivors and the churches. But to me they're just talking about the surface. There's a helluva lot more to reconcile than that. It goes much deeper. Reconciliation between members of families, between different families—the Hatfield-McCoy syndrome—and between communities and nations, Blackfoot and Cree, for example. Only then should there be talk of reconciliation with churches. But the churches are clamouring: 'Forgive us, forgive us.' They've got it all backward."

Noel is talking about colonialism and the underlying systemic problems that made the residential schools possible, or inevitable. He gives an example of how during his talks he focuses on the blondest, most blue-eyed student in a class, asking that person to consider how he or she might have felt in a similar situation, after being robbed, displaced, brainwashed, even raped, then asking, "Think what that would do to your children, your siblings, all those around you that you love. Put that on for now and think about it. When you see an Aboriginal person who's done something contrary to the laws of this country, ask yourself what might have produced that anger, that dysfunction. I've spoken to hundreds, even thousands of people about these things in the last few years. The kids understand that."

"When I address older, more sophisticated kids," he says, "I'll talk about the treaties, how promises were made on the authority of the bible on one side and the authority of traditional beliefs on the other. Those promises were broken by the Christians."

He's prepared to acknowledge that Christianity and traditional spirituality have a lot in common. "They're closer than you think," he tells the young people, "so don't disparage traditional beliefs. Those promises were made in front of God."

"I don't sugar-coat it," he tells me. "I spoke to some graduating teachers. They brought in an Elder who'd not been abused in school. Then I came in and said the opposite. Some wrote in their assessment form that Starblanket is bitter. They want to whitewash it all. I don't get that here at the university, but once I was scheduled to speak at a high school with 1,200 kids. The day I was to arrive, 250 kids called in sick. There's lots of work to be done yet."

The last thing Noel Starblanket says in the earlier Donald Brittain film, during his speech to the Saskatchewan Federation of Indian Nations, is, "I'll give you the next two years of my life." He's given more than four decades and won't be stopping soon.

nineteen

Plains Song

During my days in Regina, as the guest of my friends Bruce Rice and Joanne Havelock, I re-read James Daschuk's *Clearing the Plains: Disease, Politics of Starvation, and the Loss of Aboriginal Life*, in which he aims to "identify the roots of the current health disparity between the indigenous and mainstream populations in western Canada."[35] His is not a disinterested analysis of the conditions of the Indigenous people of the Great Plains but a passionate, well-documented indictment of government policy. He wants to identify root causes: "Health as a measure of humane experience cannot be considered in isolation from the social and economic forces that shape it. In Canada, the marginalization of First Nations people has been the primary factor impeding improved health outcomes for all of its citizens."[36] After announcing his intentions, Daschuk comes right to the point: "Racism among the policy makers and members of mainstream society was the key factor in creating the gap in health outcomes as well as maintaining a double standard for acceptable living conditions for the majority of the population."[37]

I have spent a lot of energy and stomach lining over a lifetime venting in print and in lectures about the effects of racism in Canada and abroad, seeing it as the main ingredient in the devastation of the Indigenous peoples in Canada, the Maya, the Palestinians, the tribes and nations of Africa, and so many other peoples and jurisdictions. However, after travelling to Africa and reading of that continent's colonial history, I realized I was only half right.

It's greed that drives colonization; racism just oils the wheels. The colonial project uses racism as the means of controlling the people and exploiting the resources of new territories. Joseph Conrad saw material interests as the motivating factor, with London, Paris, Brussels, Berlin, and Amsterdam as the real seats of empire, where the dark hearts could be heard beating and scheming. Daschuk understands this as well although, in *Clearing the Plains*, his main focus is on "biological warfare." He insists that "those who place human agency and greed and the expansionism of colonial powers at the centre of the decline of indigenous nations in the western hemisphere are missing half of the story; the role played by biology cannot be ignored. It was a fundamental principle in the history of indigenous America."[38]

Canada's rivers and lakes, like the highways of Africa that helped the spread of AIDS, were the principal transportation corridors for diseases. So, too, the re-introduction of horses in the Americas was another factor in the rapid spread of disease, particularly smallpox (Variola major), tuberculosis, and other pathogens such as measles and whooping cough. These diseases came with the Europeans, but their effects and spread could have been radically reduced had it not been for government parsimony fuelled by racism: "The most significant factor under human control was the failure of the Canadian government to meet its treaty obligations and its decision to use food as a means to control the Indian population to meet its development agenda rather than as a response to a humanitarian crisis."[39]

What Daschuk discovers is a "politics of famine."[40] In his highly detailed and articulate study, he reveals that economics as well as biology were responsible for most deaths:

> Yet not all First Nations endured this transitional period of hunger and sickness. The Dakota, who farmed, did not depend exclusively on the bison and were not signatories to the treaties, were able to maintain relatively good conditions in their communities. There is evidence that the emerging TB epidemic was not an organic phenomenon but the outcome of prolonged malnutrition and failure of the dominion to meet its treaty commitments.[41]

Those who believe that everything was hunky-dory, except for a few bad apples in the residential schools, should reconsider the corruption, nepotism, and abuse by government officials, Indian agents, and food contractors, who withheld rations or supplied rotten, infected, substandard food to starving First Nations. Daschuk concludes that the removal of all tribes from land south of the new railway constituted "the ethnic cleansing of southwest Saskatchewan."[42] Indigenous people starved while stores of purchased food rotted in warehouses. Prime Minister John A. Macdonald, as we have seen, bragged in Parliament about keeping the Indians on the verge of starvation, a condition that resulted in malnutrition and compromised immune systems, ripe for disease.

The report of Dr. Kittson of Fort McLeod, brought to my attention by both Lux and Daschuk, that "the people under his care were receiving less than half the ration provided to state prisoners in Siberia," is a reminder that there were doctors who knew and objected to what was happening to Indigenous people.[43] The ignoring of Kittson and the firing of a doctor such as Daniel Hagarty, whose work saved countless lives, are further evidence that white settlement and development were the driving forces, the fruits of a racist agenda marked by cynicism and indifference.

The much-touted transition of Indigenous populations from hunting-based to agriculture-based societies was never taken seriously by the government. In addition to displacing First Nations to the least arable land and the failure of promised farm equipment to arrive—or for it to be late and substandard—the program was undermined by corruption, drought, the deliberate withholding of food, the pass system, and the refusal to allow Indigenous people to sell their produce openly. Indigenous agriculture did not have a chance in the face of zoonotic diseases, including bovine TB transferred from diseased Texas cattle herds purchased by Baker, the principal supplier and contractor, who double-billed for his services, and wheeler-dealer Lieutenant-Governor Edgar Dewdney, who Daschuk believes was clearly on the take.

143

My long trek through the minefields of white–Indigenous relations and medical history certainly confirms Daschuk's analysis and suggests that we are a long way from a solution. I'm carrying with me on this trip across the country the experiences shared by Joan Morris, Belvie Brebber, Marilyn

Murray-Allison, Linda McDonald, Melinda Bullshields, and others. Fraught with racial slurs, subtle or blatant humiliations, and the constant potential for violence, the daily rituals of doing business, purchasing food, getting an education, or simply conducting life as an Indigenous person in Canada can be challenging at best. At the worst, going through life under these conditions is enough to bring on addiction, illness, and despair. A trip to the hospital for an emergency or a simple test leaves one open to racist responses, not to mention the possibility of slapdash diagnoses and treatment. The reasons for this are multiple, not least the government's determination to do as little as possible for the health and wellbeing of Indigenous peoples.

In *First Peoples, Second Class Treatment*, Billie Allan and Janet Smylie see racist stereotypes as the bedrock, or ground zero, of Indigenous health issues, and take pains to show how these stereotypes have been shaped by colonial attitudes and practice. Although admitting that the idea of race is socially constructed and has no basis in biology, they acknowledge the usefulness of this construct when it comes to the trampling of rights, theft of land, and all manner of discrimination. In addition to identifying several types of racism—including systemic, interpersonal, epistemic, and internalized—Allan and Smylie also talk about other forms of violence, including pressures that result in attempts to mask one's Indigenous identity, and the effects these can have on the individual's health:

> Pointing to the growing body of research in the US and Australia that identifies racism as a chronic stressor implicated in the health of African Americans and Indigenous Australians, the researchers argue for increased research attention to examining the contributions of racism to the persistent health disparities experienced by Indigenous peoples in Canada.[44]

Notwithstanding assumptions about the values we place on diversity, it may surprise many to learn that the rates of racial discrimination against Indigenous peoples in Canada are much higher than those experienced by Black and Latino peoples in the US.[45]

The situation may be complex, but the steps towards a solution, according to Allan and Smylie, are less so:

Understanding the impact of historic, collective and intergenerational trauma in the lives of Indigenous peoples is a necessary precondition to improving health care access and service delivery. Moreover, it is foundational to informing anti-racist efforts addressing the pathologizing and dehumanizing stereotypes that have fuelled the marginalization and poor treatment of Indigenous peoples in Canadian society, and to advancing awareness of how these stereotypes are reinforced by the ongoing social exclusion and inequities faced by Indigenous communities subsequent to these traumas, including poverty, unemployment, homelessness and poor health.[46]

Systemic racism compounded by negative stereotypes and the myth of settler innocence—root causes of Indigenous malaise and ill health—is entrenched and will not be quickly eradicated. The work requires a major

shift in how matters of racism and racialization are taken up by Canadian social institutions beyond the health care system, including education, child protection and justice, as well as how these issues are accounted for and addressed by public policies and formal legislation. It requires a departure from the cherished image of Canada as the well-meaning, international peacekeeper and the imagined harmony of the multicultural mosaic, and a long walk towards truth and reconciliation.[47]

I don't see this happening soon, as our ingrained suspicion of the Other and our apparent need for a scapegoat are being fed by vested interests of all sorts. As for the First Nations, Métis, and Inuit, their damage is profound and their hurt deep. Even Murray Sinclair, a beacon of hope and sanity, believes that full healing could take seven generations.

twenty

Birds, Not Clerics _____

C lifford Cardinal (not to be confused with Harold) is sitting across from me at the apartment of Nancy Gibson and John Whittaker, slowly stirring the cup of tea in his left hand, weighing the mood and situation in the room. We were supposed to meet three days earlier, but he hadn't shown up or responded to my emails or phone calls. Thanks to an intervention in the form of a text message from my hosts' daughter, he finally made contact. Having spent the previous week working as a healer in the foothills west of Edmonton, he's arrived late.

"Clifford, there are too many Cardinals in this story. Readers are going to get confused." I expect him to make a rude comment along the lines of "What readers?" But he's not one to go for the easy target. He takes a sip of tea and closes his eyes to savour the taste, his lips stretching into a thin smile.

"Gary, the church is lousy with cardinals, the city of St. Louis too, so why shouldn't the Cree also have a lot of them?"

I'd forgotten how tall he is—a long drink of water, as we used to say—and how quick-witted and likable. Of course, it's impossible to resist a person with a good sense of humour, which is what is making my Dantean descent through limbo and hell more bearable.

Thousands of pinpricks of light on Edmonton's Southside have come on across the North Saskatchewan River valley. In Clifford's absence, Nancy and John have been extremely solicitous, not only putting me up, and putting up with me, but also arranging encounters with three dynamic Indigenous women—forces of nature, John assures me—working at a variety of levels in the community, including the justice system and the Native Counselling Service of Alberta. We'd stopped by a new safe house or residence to meet the director, Rocky Ward, but she was not available. We were also encouraged to talk to Maggie Hodgson, whom I had first read about in *Stolen from Our Embrace*. I knew of Maggie's work as a researcher at the Nechi Institute, connected with Poundmaker's Lodge Treatment Centre, where she had so much to offer about dealing with addictions and with sexual abusers within the communities where offences took place. Unfortunately, she too was not in her office.

Two hours and several phone calls later, John's told we can find Rocky Ward at Simply Café on 124th Street, one of a network of Indigenous eating and meeting places designed to assist recovering alcoholics, help with suicide prevention, and provide general support. To our surprise, we've hit the jackpot. Not only is Rocky Ward here, but so are Maggie Hodgson, Victoria Whalen, and Sheila Courtellier, all of them having come from a special ceremony in the city. After some small talk, John leaves me to my own devices. The seating arrangement is not good and the table a bit cramped. I sit facing Rocky, with Maggie on my right, and beside her Sheila, whom I can't see at all. Victoria Whalen is seated diagonally across the table. I start from scratch, none of them having heard of me or my project, other than John's brief introduction.

I talk a bit about my work in Africa, my meeting with Joan Morris at the TRC hearings in Victoria, my encounters with former patients at the Camsell and Nanaimo Indian hospitals, and my interviews with Elders across the country. It feels a bit stilted, and I know it must sound even more so to these four women who've just had their coffee break interrupted by a complete stranger. I'm conscious of not being able to make eye contact with the two women on my right. Rocky Ward and Vicky Whalen agree to meet with me the following day. I give them each a segregated hospital brochure and the promise of a copy of *Drink the Bitter Root*. As we're about to leave, Maggie Hodgson, who has been listening carefully, especially to my comments about visiting the Camsell graves and Poundmaker's addiction centre, mentions Gitxsan Elder George Muldoe, a former student at the Edmonton Residential School in St. Albert, who had been conscripted to dig some of those graves. She also offers a caution.

"I'd like, respectfully, to give you some advice about your use of the term 'story.' A friend of mine, making his claim regarding abuse experience at the residential school, was being interviewed by a lawyer for the Anglican Church. After he'd finished, the lawyer tossed him a toonie and said: 'Buy yourself a lottery ticket. You've got about as much chance of winning the lottery as you have of getting any money out of the Anglican Church. Nice story, though.'"

Maggie does not need to explain further. The disbelief and lack of respect invested in the phrase "nice story" is not lost on me. In fact, it's something that Joanie mentioned months earlier. I'd been trying to shift to using "testimony" or "shared experience" as often as possible, but it has been difficult because, as a writer, the word "story" does not have the negative connotation for me as something false or made up. All history is someone's story, subject to the distortions of memory, the failings of the senses, and mediated by the character, experience, and ideology of the teller or sharer. I don't make the mistake of trying to explain this to Maggie but thank her for the good advice. I regret being unable to talk with her privately.

The next morning, I arrive at the Buffalo Sage Wellness House in downtown Edmonton. Actually, it is five or six houses linked together on 104 Avenue and is devoted to the "Respect and Dignity of All." Buffalo Sage is a minimum-security prison with sixteen beds for female offenders. I've done my homework and checked out the facility's website, whose preamble reminds me of the need for new attitudes and correctional alternatives:

> It is no secret that Aboriginal women are over-represented in the criminal justice system. This over-representation is even more apparent in the Prairie Region where Aboriginal women offenders are the fastest-growing population and represent over half of the women offenders in federal custody.[48]

Vicky Whalen has been described to me as the warden of this institution, but her business card describes her position as Spiritual/Cultural Advisor. We talk briefly about the challenges and high expectations she faces working in the only Indigenous women's prison in Canada, but the conversation shifts quickly to books and her mother's experience as a patient at the Camsell, where her eyes had been "peeled" in response to some sort of infection and were never quite right after that. When I mention the experiments at Goodfish Lake RC Day School, she's appalled and tells me she's heard rumours of involuntary injections at a military base in southern Alberta as well.

"One of my longstanding concerns, racist policies that discriminate against Aboriginal women," she confides, "was finally addressed in Bill C-31, giving Status rights back to Aboriginal women who married non-Status men."

Most of our brief time together is spent talking about healing. Vicky shares her experience of using role-playing sessions to educate people about what has been going on in Canadian society, where those who participate inside a rope circle as "parents," faced with the interference and aggression of those acting as Indian agents, principals, RCMP, and bureaucrats, end up literally fighting to retain possession of the stuffed animals that represent children. I'd witnessed that kind of drama therapy during a year of graduate studies in education in England and learned more about its use by field workers of the International Criminal Court in Africa to enable victims of violence to acknowledge, act out, and confront their trauma. In this case, it's being used to make settlers fully grasp what our ancestors have done to Indigenous peoples.

I tell Clifford about these women I've met in his absence to let him know I've put the time meant for him to good use, but also because I'm realizing that this is not just about him and me and Goodfish Lake. It's about something larger, about our friendship and mutual liberation, our ability to learn from and transcend the travesties of our troubled and shared history. Since my visit to Library and Archives Canada the previous week in Ottawa, which turned up nothing to confirm that the Goodfish Lake RC Day School was run as a laboratory, I've realized that Clifford and I need to alter our strategy. I'm interested in exploring the local options, in particular the files allegedly stored in Miss X's basement.

149

According to Clifford, as a teenager Miss X assisted her aunt and Ms. Ruhlhoff in recording the vaccinations administered at the Goodfish Lake RC day school. Clifford has been aware of the existence of this material for two decades, but has resisted the temptation to apply pressure for its release. After all, it does not belong to him and may have implications that will put other members of the community in harm's way, or at least cast them in a bad light. I try to convince him that Miss X would be doing the Goodfish Lake people, and the larger Indigenous community, a service in bringing to the fore any new information on the subjecting of Indigenous children to involuntary experiments, especially ones that may have had such lethal consequences.

"In my view, hers would be a heroic act. And it would certainly help to eliminate any residual guilt she might feel for having participated in those trials, however unwittingly."

Edmonton is quiet now, the hum of traffic gone. John and Nancy excused themselves an hour earlier to give us some privacy. Clifford's tired, but he lets me go on talking. However, I know enough to shut up and let him weigh the options, the long-term impacts of this exposure, on his life, Miss X's, and the lives of the Goodfish Lake Cree.

The silence that follows is comfortable, but Clifford stands up to go. "I get the message, Gary, but what I need first is a massage from Delores, who hasn't seen me for more than a week."

twenty-one

Scales of Justice _____

My meeting with Vicky Whalen and my visit to Buffalo Sage Wellness House, where we talked about alternatives to conventional corrections, set me thinking again about the inevitable link between justice and healing for Indigenous people. The former Conservative government came to power in part because of their tough-on-crime agenda, despite the fact that per-capita crime was diminishing in Canada, and judges, lawyers, and law-enforcement officers opposed more rigorous measures of punishment. The Conservatives promised to build more prisons and to impose mandatory sentences for drug offenses, sex crimes, and child exploitation. They promptly passed Bill C-10 with Senate approval, while clear indicators were emerging that a similar surge of tougher sentences and the construction of privately run prisons in the US had failed to reduce crime. In an article in *USA Today*, March 30, 2014, entitled "Toughness on Crime Gives Way to Fairness, Cost Reality," Kevin Johnson suggests that the state of New York was rethinking and retooling its prison system.

At a certain point under the direction of Governor Rockefeller, the state could not build new prisons fast enough. Now, it seems, New York is not only overwhelmed by the cost, but it is also coming to the enlightened conclusion that mandatory minimum sentences for non-violent offenders and the solitary confinement of mothers, juveniles, and the mentally ill are not only wrong-headed, but also counterproductive. Or, in the words of David Kennedy, director of the National Network for Safe Communities at John

Jay College of Criminal Justice, "What ties them all together is the basic recognition that the application of power without justice is brutal. And there is nothing democratic about brutality."[49] In short, there is nothing to recommend a system that is more punitive than educational or restorative.

While individual or collective revenge can be sweet, at least temporarily, it does not address the social problems—poverty, displacement, racism, unemployment, and lack of educational opportunity—that contribute to crime. Jail time also tends to harden convicted offenders. My thinking about these matters shifted when I was confronted with the challenging conditions in sub-Saharan Africa while researching my book *Drink the Bitter Root*. The scale of violence was so colossal in Rwanda—the murder of 800,000 Tutsis and sympathetic Hutus, including most lawyers and judges, in one hundred days—that individual justice was not only impossible, but clearly a luxury. All that was possible under the circumstances was a sort of grassroots system called *gacaca*, where perpetrators sometimes found themselves sitting as judges.

Things were not much better in the small town of Gulu in northern Uganda. As I imagined a slow, painful death for Joseph Kony and his ragtag Lord's Resistance Army, my Acholi friend Nancy wished to have those who had mutilated her and killed her friends restored to the community because they were mostly abducted boys who had been brainwashed and terrorized into becoming professional killers. I'd been told about Acholi justice, where the emphasis was not on punishment and revenge, which so often spirals out of control, but on restoring the balance in the community destroyed by a crime. This all sounded good in the abstract, but hearing it come from an actual victim touched me deeply. I decided I would try to learn more about restorative justice and healing circles back home, where an Indigenous population of about 6 per cent occupies 38 per cent of the available places in prisons.

On my return to Canada, I had the good fortune to discover John Reilly's book *Bad Medicine: A Judge's Struggle for Justice in a First Nations Community*. He describes his transition from a young hotshot judge determined to sock it to offenders, delivering justice equally to all who came before his court. Before long, he began to notice the high level of recidivism amongst Indigenous offenders, jail time seeming to have had no positive effect whatsoever. This prompted him to get to know the Stoney people in his area, where he quickly realized that some are less equal than others when it comes to their capacity to walk a straight line and to live within the law. This prompted him to ask why this was so. He also discovered section 718 in the Criminal Code, which had not come to his attention in law school, or been pointed out by other colleagues in the profession, but which would help to change the way he thought about the law and his application of it:

> The fundamental purpose of sentencing is to protect society and to contribute, along with crime prevention initiatives, to respect for the law and the maintenance of a just, peaceful and safe society by imposing just sanctions . . . 718.2 (e) all available sanctions, other than imprisonment, that are reasonable in the circumstances . . . should be considered for all offenders, with particular attention to the circumstances of Aboriginal offenders.[50]

This section, unnoticed or ignored at the time by most judges and lawyers, confirmed Reilly's feeling that a different, more humane approach to Indigenous offenders was needed. Taking into account the historical realities—displacement, the Indian Act, racism, and residential schools for starters—he began to recommend restorative justice alternatives, healing circles, and counselling instead of hard time. His approach was met with criticism from bureaucrats and colleagues who considered him "soft on Indians." Although he was aware that serious offenders needed to be put out of circulation, he also realized that the system needed to make it easier for minor offenders to be reformed and restored to the community. However, it was also clear that the corrections system in Canada, overburdened with Indigenous offenders, many of them poor and suffering from addictions or mental illnesses, almost all of them victims of intergenerational trauma, needed to shift its focus from punishment to restoration, turning the wayward and the lost, with their untapped human potential, into productive individuals.

It's been a long time coming, but an indication that this message is being heard can be seen on the website of Correctional Service Canada under the heading "Restorative Justice—A Worthy Approach":

153

Restorative Justice (RJ) helps meet the needs of people faced with crime and conflict in an inclusive and meaningful way. RJ practices provide voluntary opportunities for those who have been harmed and those who have caused harm to be active participants in their journey for justice, accountability, and reparation.

CSC supports the advancement of RJ as it contributes to CSC's priorities and public safety. In addition to CSC's most reputable work in providing victim-offender mediation services, RJ approaches are used to develop collaborative partnerships, address conflict, and assist offenders in their exploration of RJ values and principles.[51]

If the Gladue Report, the Official Apology, and the TRC's final report can't convince Canadians of the need for special treatment, and a re-thinking of our relations with Indigenous peoples, perhaps the final speech of Levi General will. Otherwise known as Deskaheh, this great Iroquois (Haudenosaunee) chief travelled to Geneva to file grievances at the League of Nations in 1923 after the Canadian government dissolved the traditional governing council of the Six Nations Confederacy. It's a painfully witty and eloquent reminder that there are plenty of good reasons for Indigenous peoples to have little respect for Canadian law and so-called justice. Here are a few excerpts from his radio address, delivered a few weeks before he died in 1925, in exile across the border in Rochester, New York:

> Nearly everyone who is listening to me is a pale face, I suppose. I am not. My skin is not red but that is what my people are called by others. My skin is brown, light brown, but our cheeks have a little flush and that is why we are called red skins. We don't mind that. There is no difference between us, under the skins, that any expert with a carving knife has ever discovered.
>
> My home is on the Grand River. Until we sold off a large part, our country extended down to Lake Erie, where, 140 winters ago, we had a little sea-shore of our own and a birch-bark navy. You would call it Canada. We do not. We call the little ten-miles square we have left the "Grand River Country." We have the right

to do that. It is ours. We have the written pledge of George III that we should have it forever as against him or his successors and he promised to protect us in it.

We didn't think we would ever live long enough to find that a British promise was not good. An enemy's foot is on our country, and George V knows it for I told him so, but he will not lift his finger to protect us nor will any of his ministers. One who would take away our rights is, of course, our enemy . . .

In some respects, we are just like you. We like to tell our troubles. You do that. You told us you were in great trouble a few winters ago because a great big giant with a big stick was after you. We helped you whip him. Many of our young men volunteered and many gave their lives for you. You were very willing to let them fight in the front ranks in France. Now we want to tell our troubles to you.

I do not mean that we are calling on your governments—we are tired of calling on the governments of pale-faced peoples in America and in Europe. We have tried that and found it was no use. They deal only in fine words—we want something more than that. We want justice from now on. After all that has happened to us, that is not too much to ask. You got half of your territory here by warfare upon redmen, usually unprovoked, and you got about a quarter of it by bribing their chiefs, and not over a quarter of it did you get openly and fairly. You might have gotten a good share of it by fair means if you had tried.[52]

In what follows, Deskaheh makes the point that the Canadian justice system does not operate equally for all people, suggesting that those with money, power, and influence can usually avoid incarceration. While attacking British imperialism, he is not averse to making a wise-crack about high levels of corruption in Canadian society and government. He reminds listeners not only that his own people practice justice without jails and are mostly unfamiliar with treachery and lies, but also that they fought alongside us in the Great War but were treated like dirt when they returned, losing rights and property.

When Ottawa tried that, our people resented it. We knew that would mean the end of our government. Because we did so, the Canadian Government began to enforce all sorts of Dominion and Provincial laws over us and quartered armed men among us to enforce Canadian laws and customs upon us . . .

To punish us for trying to preserve our rights, the Canadian Government has now pretended to abolish our government by Royal Proclamation, and has pretended to set up a Canadian-made government over us, composed of the few traitors among us who are willing to accept pay from Ottawa and do its bidding. Finally, Ottawa officials, under pretence of a friendly visit, asked to inspect our precious wampum belts, made by our Fathers centuries ago as records of our history, and when shown to them, these false-faced officials seized and carried away those belts as bandits take away your precious belongings. The only difference was that our aged wampum-keeper did not put up his hands—our hands go up only when we address the Great Spirit. Yours go up, I hear, only when some one of you is going through the pockets of his own white brother. According to your newspapers, they are up now a good deal of the time.

The Ottawa government thought that with no wampum belts to read in the opening of our Six Nations Councils, we would give up our home rule and self-government, the victims of superstition. Any superstition of which the Grand River People have been victims is not in reverence for wampum belts, but in their trust in the honor of governments who boast of a higher civilization.

twenty-two

Itching for Change

Lorraine Yuzicapi lives at the end of a long dirt road on the Standing Buffalo reserve, north of Fort Qu'Appelle, Saskatchewan. It takes some complicated directions to find the place: "Go up the east side of Echo Lake past Fort San, turn right at the stop sign, go up the hill to the intersection, and turn left, go for a mile or so until you come to the silos and the house with the two old school buses rusting in the yard, then turn left and follow the curve to the end of the road where you'll find a white house."

I never did see the old chapel on the left I was supposed to notice along the way. However, I flagged down an oncoming vehicle to make sure I was going in the right direction. To my surprise, Lorraine was waiting for me at the door, thanks not to intuition or smoke signals, but to a cell-phone call from that friendly mini-van, a sign that people out here look after each other.

When it was suggested that I contact Lorraine, I looked her up on the Internet, where her traditional foods booklet has been reproduced. Lorraine is Dakota, but her mother and grandmothers came from Wood Mountain Lakota Nation, sometimes referred to as Hunkpapi, or the Sitting Bull people. She explains that the Sioux Nation is divided into seven sacred campfires and each one has different ways of preparing food. Hers is the way of her mother and grandmothers, the legacy a gift for listening and watching how food is gathered, prepared, and stored. Her great-grandmother, who lived to be 107, was not only passionate about foods, but was also an excellent teacher.

157

When I first spoke to Lorraine on her cell, she sounded a bit hesitant, but as soon as I mentioned Gary Bosgoed and Noel Starblanket, she chuckled and asked me to call back on her home phone. She was community health rep for twenty years for the Standing Buffalo people, she said, and after witnessing a diabetes amputation she began to study the disease and its causes, which she attributes to chemicals, lack of exercise, and bad food choices. As one of thirteen children raised on a traditional diet, she helped her family survive by gathering, gardening, hunting, and fishing.

"Last week I made a rosehip berry pudding. Tomorrow, my whole family will come by for wild rice soup and roasted elk sandwiches." Although she lost her husband to cancer in 2000 and had the dubious distinction of being one of a tiny minority to go almost blind from the medication she took for breast cancer, she survived to become a popular guest at powwows and conferences worldwide, speaking on how to gather, prepare, and preserve traditional foods.

"A man came to one of my talks in the States. He was 250 pounds. When he came back the following year, after following my advice, he was 160 pounds. All his friends thought he was sick. Not sick, just healthy."

Lorraine has a section and a half (almost a thousand acres) connected with the reserve on which she and her family have always gathered the plants and herbs required for a traditional diet. Now that she is legally blind, with barely 40 per cent vision in one eye, her friends and kids do the gathering. She persuaded the band to declare it a cultural heritage site, to be protected long term.

"My sons all hunt and fish, as well as doing their full-time jobs. My daughters do nature art, using dried fish scales and porcupine quills, for example. I clean and preserve in the traditional way. Nothing is wasted," she tells me. "Even fish guts can be used for tanning hides, making them soft, but it takes time, which not everyone has."

To my surprise, her sons hunt elk and buffalo. Apparently, there is a nearby valley where buffalo are raised by the First Nation and available to families and for community feasts.

All this information comes to me over the phone from a woman who loves her chosen work and enjoys sharing the information. As the tribes have common foods, but quite different preparations, she spends a lot of time sharing and learning. She tells me she's not a healer, but more of a traditional nutritionist.

"Take honey, for example," she says. "It's good for colds. It takes longer but does not create immunities from overuse as antibiotics do. Just dilute and drink twice a day; it's good for arthritis too."

I ask if I can visit her on my cross-Canada trip in the fall.

"Let me know the dates well in advance," she says, "as I may be on the road. I go to Manitoulin every year. They seem to like what I have to say about foods." Then she tells me about preparing wild hazelnuts for fish or duck pemmican. "A chunk of pemmican the size of a golf ball is sufficient protein for the day. As for rosehips, soak them in hot water, then mash. A spoonful of the pulp per day will clear up the esophagus and intestines," she says with a laugh. "But not too much or the little hairs that do the cleaning will give you an itchy anus."

When I arrive at her house, it's not my anus that is itchy, but my curiosity. Lorraine has warned me in advance that the kitchen is being renovated and the house is in chaos. So I'm not surprised to find her standing behind a combination bookshelf and cabinet in the middle of the room, as if tending bar. There is a blanket on the wall, one of her specialties, covered with stars, and a couple of boxes overflowing with sweetgrass, which she sends to a First Nation in Ontario in exchange for cedar. She's proud of the ground-level addition her husband arranged to be built before he died, which he supervised from his wheelchair in the elevated kitchen. It's useful for those large family gatherings, where her kids and grandchildren can't wait to indulge in Lorraine's traditional meals.

I've brought Lorraine a copy of *Drink the Bitter Root*, hardly appropriate given the condition of her eyes; some smoked salmon from the west coast; and a packet of Virginia Shag tobacco from a small shop in Regina. We talk a lot about traditional foods, practices and values as the path back to physical and mental health for Indigenous people. There's no shortage of examples, she assures me, but weaning her people off cheap, easily accessible processed food is the problem.

159

"It takes time and effort, all that cleaning and processing. After the hunt, hours of butchering, smoking, and packaging. Not everyone has the time, or wants to spend the time, when the alternatives are so handy. Especially for those who live in town."

I wonder how much wild game there is available, especially if all the Indigenous people on reserves were to make the shift to traditional foods. Domesticating buffalo is not difficult. The problem would be to do that and raise plants without the pesticides and fertilizer chemicals that are now poisoning the environment, including nearby Echo Lake. As for numbers, the fires in northern Saskatchewan have driven dear, bear, and elk south to the point that they have become a problem for local farmers.

"How is that?" I ask.

"The elk not only eat the hay bales, but urinate around them and the cows won't touch what's left. The smell puts them off."

A month earlier, her sons and other men at Standing Buffalo were hired by farmers in the southwest of the province to hunt elk that had invaded the area.

It would be difficult to overestimate the importance of traditional foods in restoring the health of Indigenous peoples and rebuilding their connection to culture and the land. Nancy J. Turner, an ethnobotanist and professor at the University of Victoria, has written extensively on the subject of Indigenous cultivation, harvesting, and preparation of native plants. In 2008 she co-authored an article with Katherine L. Turner, published in the journal *Botany*, and titled, "Where Our Women Used to Get the Food: Cumulative Effects and Loss of Ethnobotanical Knowledge and Practice; Case Study from Coastal British Columbia." It's an important, timely, and clear analysis of the many causes and long-term impacts of colonization on Indigenous health, tracing the gradual demise of native plant harvesting and use by BC's First Nations and the long-time effects of this profound dietary shift on Indigenous health. She quotes several people from the Tsawataineuk community in Kingcome Inlet, including Hereditary Chief Cesaholis addressing the Royal Commission on Indian Affairs for the Province of BC, June 4, 1914:

> At the mouth of our river on both sides . . . a man by the name of McKay came to build his house on that place . . . This McKay took for himself the land where our forefathers always got their food . . .

where the women used to take the roots out of the ground . . . They put down stakes [to] mark the boundary lines for each one, and to our surprise this whiteman came and just took the place and . . . our women were surprised to be ordered away from that place and they don't know why they were ordered away . . . [The women] persisted to go to that place to get the food. Each woman had a wooden spade and a basket. The spade was to take up the roots, and the basket was to carry the roots, and these were taken from them and thrown away by this whiteman, and this whiteman he immediately put a fence around the place enclosing the place where our women used to get the food, and for the first time then we come to know the troubles that we are in now in our own land, and when the food of my people grew on that place.[53]

Add cattle and pigs to this mix and you can imagine how quickly the traditional plants, along with the peoples' spirits and harvesting practices, withered and died.

After discussing the importance of five traditional foods—camas, springbank clover, edible seaweed, Pacific crabapple, and thimbleberry shoots—the Turners discuss the devastating effects of colonial policies on Indigenous "health and cultural integrity."[54] Land seizures, industrial development, cattle farming, pressures to join the wage economy, pollution, habitat destruction, laws banning traditional gathering and food sharing, all served to destroy the knowledge, solidarity, and celebration around food. High rates of poverty amongst Indigenous people mean that many are still dependent on the least nutritious elements in the modern Western diet. This includes excessive carbohydrates and sugars and low-nutritional packaged foods, which have led to devastating rates of obesity, heart problems, and type 2 diabetes far above the national averages.

On a positive note, the Turners end their article with examples of this trend being reversed, at least for a few in non-urban settings:

Some Indigenous people, like Lekwungen (Songhees) Lands Manager Cheryl Bryce, regard the re-adoption of traditional foodstuffs as a way to combat some of the health problems such as diabetes facing indigenous populations today. They also see

rebuilding food sovereignty as an important step in the struggle
to overcome some of the most negative socio-cultural impacts of
colonialism.[55]

Lorraine's time with me is limited. She's spent the previous day at a Treaty 4
event talking to seven hundred people in small groups that passed through
her tent to learn about traditional foods. The challenge, she explains, was
having to constantly shift her delivery to accommodate the different age
groups, from small children to teenagers to adults. It was an exhausting
procession, but one she would not give up willingly. Now the phone is ringing with people who will be dropping by to visit and pick up her special
foods and traditional medicines. She won't let me go without giving me a
few strips of elk pemmican for the road. As we've talked about our children
intermittently, Lorraine mentions a daughter who works as an RCMP officer in Beausejour, Manitoba. I tell her I'll try to call to say hello when I'm
in the same small town in a few weeks to see my ageing stepmother.

The road back is easier, substituting the lefts for right turns, until I
come to the road that will take me south past the legendary but now abandoned tuberculosis sanatorium at Fort San.

twenty-three

Fort Qu'Appelle

As I drive south along the eastern shore of Echo Lake towards Fort San, my mind is awash with memories of my adult links with Saskatchewan, including readings, poetry workshops, literary festivals, and many contacts with writers. The friends I made during my early years as a writer have remained important to me. I'd found the Prairies to be a healthy and nourishing milieu for writing. The solidarity and collective spirit that created the Co-operative Commonwealth Federation (CCF), the socialist party that would eventually morph into the NDP, seemed to have imbued the writers here with a rare sense of engagement and community. There was little of the star system operating elsewhere in Canada and abroad, just a sense that each writer, in however large or small a way, was contributing to the greater text that would be left behind as a testimony to the prairie, its peoples, and their times.

James Daschuk, whose work I admire, is evidence that the tradition continues. We met recently for the first time at the Saskatchewan Writers Festival in Moose Jaw where we were both participants, James reading from his much lauded non-fiction work, *Clearing the Plains*. In terms of research, James has his finger on the pulse of Canada's treatment of Indigenous peoples, so I was happy to oblige when he invited me to visit him in Regina a few days after the event. We met for lunch at La Cucaracha, a small seasonal canteen with picnic benches under a tarpaulin on 13th Avenue, to talk about our shared interests in Indigenous affairs. Having heard about my project, he was intent on a small educational mission on my behalf.

A light rain, after weeks of drought, has begun to fall when we turn off the paved highway onto the gravel road leading to the site of the former Regina Indian Industrial School, a precursor of the residential schools. It had opened in the 1890s to prepare Indigenous children for the lower levels of the white workforce, and in the 1930s it was turned into a detention centre for wayward youth, one of whom would eventually burn the building down. In its place I can see in the distance the red bricks and roof of a more modern correctional centre. Rather than take me to the actual site, Jim has other plans. He points to a small fenced area off to the right and slows the van down.

We stop beside a freshly painted white fence surrounding a small rectangular enclosure about fifty by seventy feet, the uncut grass interrupted only by two shrubs at the front right and a scrub tree at the back left. This isolated compound in a field designated for suburban development on the edge of Regina, Jim explains, is sacred ground, a graveyard for approximately twenty-eight children who died at the Regina Indian Industrial School. No digging had taken place, but sounding equipment has detected the tell-tale narrow disturbances at a certain depth in the soil indicating human remains. No crosses or markers for individual Indigenous children are to be found in the tall grass. However, beneath the scrub trees at the back of the cemetery, an elaborate carved headstone, half submerged in the soil, reveals the names John Meredith, age five, and Robert Duncan, age fifteen months, two sons of the school's first principal, A.J. McLeod. It is a grim reminder of white privilege, but also of the fact that disease and death play no favourites. Even more telling are the stuffed animals and children's paraphernalia attached to the white fence rails surrounding the cemetery.

On the right-hand gatepost, a rather weathered stuffed woolly lamb contemplates the light rain a foot or two above the exotic orange blossom of a bird of paradise. On the left a white pillowcase announces in bold caps, WE LOVE OUR CHILDREN; below it, the handwritten words, AND WE WILL ALWAYS REMEMBER. At each corner of this cotton sign, little stuffed animals—a pig, a cat, another lamb, and a tattered giraffe—the prairie equivalent of the putti, or cherubs, that once decorated tombs of the rich and can still be seen in classical art—bear witness, little companions for the afterlife, reminders that spirits continue to watch over us. Given the unruly state of the graveyard, and the absence of Indigenous names, it may seem at first glance that the spirits are on strike, but these little creatures tell another story.

That afternoon spent with Jim reminds me, even here in the car with afternoon sun reflecting off Echo Lake, that hospitals and graveyards are far too often linked in my deliberations about Indigenous health. I follow the contours of Echo Lake south, where I've arranged an interview with Gail Boehme, director of the All Nations' Healing Hospital, tucked away in the lush Qu'Appelle Valley. I recall an earlier visit to the remains of the Fort Qu'Appelle Indian Hospital on the western shore, the single smoke stack, a thrusting, phallic reminder of the limits of white supremacy. Unfortunately, this was neither Custer's nor John A. Macdonald's Last Stand, as the west and north shores of Echo Lake were chock-a-block with the manicured waterfront properties of well-to-do white settlers. The east side of the lake, by contrast, contains the cheap, makeshift housing provided by Indigenous and Northern Affairs for the members of Standing Buffalo First Nation.

I can't resist stopping farther along the shore for a nostalgic return to the grounds of Fort San—not the village that has grown up nearby, but the notorious TB sanatorium by the same name. There is hardly a family in Saskatchewan that does not have a relative or close friend who died or was a patient in this secluded but idyllic location, where medicines were few but the prescribed sunshine and bed rest were almost guaranteed. In its later years, the once exclusively white institution designated a small space for Indigenous patients, who were tolerated but not exactly welcome. The hospital opened in 1917 and had a capacity of 358 patients, for many a one-way trip. Eventually, it closed and became home to the Saskatchewan Summer School for the Arts from 1967 to 1991.

I was a guest speaker here one summer in the 1970s and spent two weeks the following year conducting a poetry workshop for a number of talented young hopefuls who would become significant names in the fields of poetry and publishing. I don't recall where we slept, whether it was over the morgue or in one of the former nurses' residences. Now the grounds, though still beautiful, are unkempt, the buildings boarded up, and the ghosts of those who'd died, so I was informed by a neighbour up the road, have persisted in staying on.

None of those ghosts take the least interest in me as I park my rental car, step over the chain and a sign warning that trespassers will be prosecuted, and wander up the curved road to the main hospital building, camera in hand. Suddenly, I hear two voices behind me. I'd seen a black pickup turn into the grounds, but had paid little notice, its two occupants now materializing in the road as I focus on some wild flowers and crumbling brickwork. One of them carries a clipboard.

"Hi, what brings you two gentlemen here?" I ask.

"We could ask the same question of you," the plumper of the two replies with more than a note of sarcasm.

Glad to oblige, I launch into an abbreviated version of my work on Indian hospitals and my Fort San teaching experience. The raised eyebrows and sceptical expressions ease somewhat and Clipboard admits to being a real estate agent showing the property to a potential developer, an interesting prospect given the location, the view, and approximately 180 treed acres. To my over-charged synapses, real estate agents, like Indian agents, seem part of the same old game of dispossession and take-over James Daschuk describes so well in *Clearing the Plains*. When I mention the number of reluctant Indigenous patients who'd died there, Clipboard informs me that even more whites had died at Fort San. I refrain from stating the obvious, that the ratio of deaths to overall population numbers tells a different story, and that you are much more susceptible to disease when displaced, starved, humiliated and, with a weakened immune system, consigned to the basement of the institution. Instead, I ask what will be required to restore the place and its buildings. I'm really imagining First Nations reclaiming or buying it, not what these two have in mind.

"Vision and deep pockets," Clipboard says with a laugh.

"Well," I can't resist adding as I turn to go, "at least there's no charge for the ghosts."

Stories emerging from the Fort San sanatorium are, to say the least, troubling, particularly that of Walter Budd from Pemmican Portage, who spent four years in the children's ward, where he experienced sexual abuse and was one of many children used as guinea pigs in drug trials. According to Budd, the nurses and orderlies were given to humiliating the young boys by making them expose themselves and fondle each other.[56] The sanitorium's predecessor, the Fort Qu'Appelle Indian Hospital, has an equally check-ered reputation. Starting in 1927, its director Dr. Robert George Ferguson was authorized to conduct BCG vaccination trials on 609 infants and newborns, a fifth of whom died before reaching age five. While it would be easy to blame these deaths on Ferguson, Maureen Lux suggests that the primary cause of so many deaths was poverty and its related illnesses, including pneumonia and gastro-intestinal disease. However, by January 1931, Ferguson was showing signs of caution, perhaps as a result of simi-lar trials in Lubeck, Germany, that had resulted in 71 deaths out of 249 vaccinated infants. A whiff of possible litigation was definitely in the air. Although the BCG trials were done with government and National Research Council approval, Ferguson was sufficiently aware of the legal implications of the study to advise, in a letter uncovered by Lux, that it was "unwise to initiate human experimental work among Indian children who are the direct wards of the government, and for which reason they are not in a position to exercise voluntary cooperation." I find it difficult to ignore the significance of his belief that Indigenous people were primitive and less evolved and thus, by implication, fair game for such trials.[57]

Whether any of these deaths were directly attributable to the BCG trials is open to debate, but there is no doubt that the attention given to the trials was at the expense of the general health of nearby communi-ties and in line with the government's refusal to address the social and political causes of disease: displacement, hunger, and the stress caused by racist policies and attitudes. Repeatedly referring to the disease as "Indian tuberculosis," a common practice among bureaucrats and the medical pro-fessionals in the Canadian Tuberculosis Association, was tantamount to racial profiling, and indeed pathologized the very notion of Indianness.

For Walter Budd, separation from family, physical and sexual abuse, and painful medical interventions contributed to an unsettled life. Having been taught little during those years, his grade four education did not serve him well in the search for work. He recovered from tuberculosis, but had continuing health problems. He's recorded in *Eagle Feather News* as saying, "I was badly scarred . . . They did a number on me."[58]

In the same issue of the magazine, celebrated novelist Richard Wagamese acknowledges the need to have these experiences recorded, made part of

167

the national narrative: "It's been a story of generations of abducted children, intergenerational pain and wounds passed down because the whole story has not been told." Wagamese insists that the truth is essential for healing, not just for victims but for the nation: "First Nations people know that. It's time that Canada came to understand the nature of that truth as well."[59]

After a quick lunch at the Valley Bakery and Café in Fort Qu'Appelle, I head to the All Nations' Healing Hospital clutching a book and a small offering of butter tarts for Gail Boehme. A charming woman, fiercely devoted to her work, Gail gives me more than an hour of her time, describing the facilities, which include thirteen acute care beds, a palliative care room, support for outpatients and diagnostic services, and a spacious maternity room with a fibreglass birthing tub. She speaks of the challenges of hiring and finances, her dreams for the hospital, and her own sensitivity training in Indigenous culture, which involved an immersion in traditional music, dance, contact with Elders, and a mind-altering experience in the sweat lodge. My tour of the facilities concludes with an introduction to Rick Favel, a traditional knowledge keeper and Elder-in-residence at the White Raven Healing Centre, a section of the hospital devoted to a coordinated Indigenous approach to mind, body, spirit, and community.

Rick steers me into the ceremonial room, where instruction and smudging take place, along with small official gatherings and mourning sessions where the bereaved can commune with the departing spirit of a loved one. He wants me to know that what takes place here is not just rituals or ceremonies, but "spiritual instruction and oral education." Then he takes me to the medicine room and talks about the harvesting and use of sweetgrass, cedar, and various traditional herbal medicines.

"White people use this too, but they add chemicals," Rick says disapprovingly, holding up a few sprigs of echinacea, a common prairie plant.

I'm interested in Rick's role at the hospital and his comment about the protocol and politics of traditional medicine.

"Although I've studied these plants and medicines for forty-five years, I'm not allowed to prescribe them," he says. "I have to send patients to healers who prescribe and send the patients back to me."

His remarks about traditional medicine remind me of the comments of Gitxsan Elder George Muldoe, who attended the Edmonton Indian

Residential School and also spent a few weeks in the Miller Bay Indian Hospital in Prince Rupert with TB. When I asked why his stay there was so short, he said it was mostly because of traditional medicines, that he was taking a mixture of hemlock, balsam, and devil's club, but mostly the latter. He practiced with traditional medicines and claimed to have had successes treating cancer, arthritis, and Parkinson's using Gonza Tea (tea tree oil) and a medicine made from the growths or deformities known as burls that grow on birch trees. In medicine, as in horticulture, perspective is everything.

Our final stop in the White Raven Healing Centre is a large, cedar-lined room with benches around the perimeter and a sweat lodge in the middle. Rick opens the door to show me the rock pile, a supply of large, rounded stones to be heated and placed in a pit inside the sweat lodge. I am thinking how this procedure resembled what I know as the traditional Scandinavian sauna, when Rick, as if reading my mind, launches into a story about being asked in Norway if he was a real Indian and then invited to a sauna in the countryside not far from Oslo. He arrived to find his host dressed in a white robe and wearing a pointed white hood. Suppressing a wave of anxiety that he'd been lured into a European branch of the Ku Klux Klan, he entered the sauna, where everyone, including the host, was in the process of disrobing.

"When in Norway," Rick laughs, pausing to light a cigarette. "So I dropped my drawers."

Another wave of anxiety washed over him when he was instructed to lie face down on what was either a simple bench or a sacrificial altar. Complying hesitantly, he was whipped lightly on the back with cedar branches, the needles creating a not entirely unpleasant prickling sensation. Told to roll over, he covered his genitals, much to the amusement of the sweating Norwegians. The whipping continued for a few minutes. Then two large, very naked bruisers each grabbed an arm, propelling him to his feet, out the door of the sauna, and down a slope full-tilt through the bushes until he found himself in mid-air—like Wile E. Coyote but without the requisite pause to recognize the gravity of the situation—then plunging down immediately into cold water, the three of them shrieking and laughing at the shock.

"We do that too, here in the snow, but not in the buff," Rick informs me, opening the second of the double doors to release the smoke from his cigarette. This is, after all, still a hospital.

169

twenty-four

Here's the Scoop

Manitoba figures prominently in Canada's Indigenous history, not only for the Louis Riel and Red River Resistance of 1870 and the Northwest Rebellion of 1885, led by Métis military leader Gabriel Dumont, but also more recently for the notoriety of MLA Elijah Harper. Born in 1949 at Red Sucker Lake Reserve in northern Manitoba, Harper was a residential school survivor and a graduate of the University of Manitoba. His fame, like that of Riel, had to do with his stand against injustice and encroachment on Indigenous rights and freedoms. When he held up an eagle feather in the provincial legislature and refused to ratify the Meech Lake Accord on the grounds that it had been negotiated with no input from Indigenous leaders, Elijah Harper changed the political dynamic in this country permanently.

Although I knew little of the region's Indigenous people, my first encounter with them was very personal. While doing research for my doctoral thesis at the London Library in 1971, I took a month off to travel in Europe and North Africa. In Morocco, I received a telegram informing me that my brother Jim Geddes had adopted two boys: Mel, whose Cree name was Deer, or Wêpâyôs, and Fred, whose Saultaux name was Rabbit Skin, or Waboozwyaan. The boys, who were half-brothers, had apparently suffered neglect and abuse in their former foster home. Without understanding any of the long-term ramifications of what we now refer to as the Sixties Scoop, this struck me as a wonderful expansion of my world. I could not wait to meet my new nephews.

Although the boys were good-natured and appeared to settle happily into their new home, their lives began to unravel during the teen years, as racism, peer pressure, and lack of confidence led them to experiment with drugs and alcohol, which resulted in a number of run-ins with the law. Their downward spiral was heart-breaking. Fred was killed when the car he was driving without a seatbelt flipped on a gravel road pinning him underneath, and Mel ended up in a wheelchair with both legs amputated, eventually dying from diabetes as a result of alcoholism and a bad diet.

Jim would later adopt two more boys. Henry, who had suffered from fetal alcohol poisoning and been a glue sniffer as a child, would die from a blow received in a Winnipeg bar. Norman, thankfully alive and well, is married and living with his wife and son in Saskatoon. Even before I learned anything about the Sixties Scoop, I could not help but feel that my family and my country had failed those boys.

My first interview on the subject of Indigenous health in Manitoba was with Eleanor James-Robertson, a Métis woman who had sent me an email describing her open-heart surgery in Winnipeg. She did not recall many details, but believed that her surgery had taken place when she was nine years old, in 1960. Later she searched the Archives of Manitoba in Winnipeg for her hospital records because she had been told she was the first child in Manitoba to have this surgery. The archives, however, indicated that a boy from Winnipeg had been the first, in 1963. She was surprised by this news, but took it in stride.

I asked her if she thought preliminary tests had been done on Indigenous children, mentioning what I'd learned thus far about First Nations, Metis, and Inuit children being used as guinea pigs. It was probably a curmudgeonly response to her email, but Eleanor responded openly and positively:

Yes, I do believe that I was a guinea pig, but I have survived! Children died before me and after me, I feel blessed. My cardiologist is now about 85 years old, Dr. Gordon Cummings, and I heard he was still practicing part time in downtown Winnipeg. I really don't know the surgeon's name, maybe Dr. Fergusson. I have always had a great relationship with Dr. Cummings who I stopped seeing when I was 27, he transferred me into adult care at that time. Maybe I was his first success!

I am trying hard to remember my mom's stories about her sister, Christina. I do know that it was a major loss for the whole family. She kept a picture of her and nobody has that picture anymore! She was a true beauty. It is quite sad how many aboriginal people died in these institutions without any care for the families who lost loved ones. They believed that we were savages, so "what is another loss[?]"

As Eleanor would explain to me later in more detail, her maternal aunt Christina Grieves was sent to Ninette Sanatorium, apparently with TB, at age 15 and died a year later. Eleanor's grandparents were never contacted and kept waiting for news. All the family knows, even today, is that there is a *"big mount outside the hospital, where the Aboriginals were buried."* Such losses were far too common, but even worse is the thought that they might have resulted from neglect or a botched operation. For Eleanor, this was just one of the many difficulties she faced.

Since I was Métis, without treaty status, I believe that I was kept in foster homes and possibly went into care with Children's Aid Society. I had a social worker all the time. The foster homes were a horror at times and all very lonely. My parents did not see me for years, because they could not afford to travel to see me. I had a paternal aunt who came to see me a few times, but I did not know her well. I did travel to Norway House on good weather days and when I was feeling healthy, those were great times. When I married, I married into treaty, so I became first nations then.

I was thinking about your wife's books, does she write fiction? Romance novels? . . . I have read Ann Rule's books, as she writes about domestic violence. This has been a big part of my marriage, which taught me to be extra careful! My husband died in 2001, but we had [been] divorced since 1983. I have done some writing, but have been scared to let it go into print. My children and I have been in a shelter at least four times. This part of my life has had a great impact in my everyday life and I doubly feel like a true survivor. I feel like a true survivor!

Geez, I have said a lot. You have become a true outlet!

Eleanor went on to say that she has suffered a lot in her personal relationships, and in her past she has resorted to hiding her emotions. This is a common trait amongst people who have lived through neglect and abuse in residential school and foster homes:

My way of coping with death or the loss of a loved one has never been the same as anyone else. I cannot cry. I remember my father's death, I felt a numbness and I had to take control of my physical self and be extra careful not to show any sign of grief or shock. I was always so centered on controlling my feelings and because of this, people have known me to be distant or non-accommodating. I have been hurt many times because I have been told that I don't care or that I'm stuck up!

When Eleanor and I finally meet in person in Winnipeg some time later, it is a brief visit punctuated by Eleanor's family concerns. She warned me in advance that she might not be at her best. Her six-year-old granddaughter and ten-week-old grandson are staying with her while their house, which sustained damage in the flood that overwhelmed Calgary earlier in the year, is being restored. It's a strange coincidence, as my Winnipeg cousins spent the summer with me on our farm in Saskatchewan during the Winnipeg flood of 1952.

Despite her stressful situation, I find Eleanor to be an open and sympathetic host, something I should have expected from the tone of her earlier emails, where she spoke of how being a social worker and case manager with young people in distress had opened her "eyes, mind, and heart" and enabled her to "see things differently." During our visit, I give her some brochures and a copy of *Kingdom of Ten Thousand Things*, even though she scarcely has enough time to read these days.

Despite her many troubles, including a Christian sister who berates her for smudging, Eleanor sends the PDF of my Indian hospital brochure to her friends and relatives across the province. Her cousin Albert McLeod responds quickly, recommending that I read Heather Robertson's *Reservations Are for Indians* and sending me the link to a recent article in the *Winnipeg Free Press* by Catherine Mitchell about a plane that crashed in bad weather on August 21, 1949, en route from Chesterfield Inlet to Winnipeg. Twenty-four people had been killed, including thirteen kabloona (white people)—seven RCAF crew, four weather station employees, a physio-therapist, and a newsman—and eleven Inuit polio victims who were being sent to the King George Hospital. It's a heart-rending story, especially for the Inuit families, who had been told that the bodies of their loved ones were too burned to be recognizable and had been buried in an unmarked common grave on the Norway House reserve.

Mitchell's story focuses on one of the Inuit victims, twelve-year-old Ubluriak ("star" in Inuktitut), and reveals that there had in fact been no fire when the Canso crashed. Although the families of the white victims were informed and the bodies of their loved ones shipped home to rela-tives, the Inuit families had been lied to: they received neither telegrams nor the bodies of loved ones. It took fifty-seven years for the real story to be told.[60]

Important historical moments from Winnipeg—the Gateway to the West—and from Manitoba generally are not in short supply, from the rebel-lions to the untimely death of Brian Sinclair, left unattended in a Winnipeg emergency room for thirty-four hours in 2008. Indeed, Westerners might call this province the Gateway to Indigenous Grief.

Such continual lies, betrayals, and withholding of information at the political, bureaucratic, and personal level have made it difficult, if not impossible, for many Indigenous peoples to trust anything said by newcomers. Stories keep surfacing which show that the seemingly harsh assessments of Harold Cardinal, Kim Recalma-Clutesi, Noel Starblanket, Levi General, Eleanor James-Robertson, and so many others are, if any-thing, understatements. Without truth being told, and inscribed in the country's permanent record, reconciliation is only a pipe-dream.

twenty-five

Without Reservation

T aking Albert McLeod's advice, I ordered a copy of Heather Robertson's *Reservations Are for Indians*, originally published in 1970. Although my interviews had given me plenty of food for thought on the effects of treaties and residential schools, I was not ready for the raw and bitter portrait Robertson paints of life at Norway House, north of Lake Winnipeg, and her strong indictment of Canada's so-called Indian policy. I had not expected such straight talk from a white journalist over four decades ago.

While waiting for the book to arrive, I had time to reflect yet again on my position as a non-Indigenous person writing about Indigenous issues. Early on in my research into the links between residential schools and Indian hospitals, I encountered a disturbing quotation by Verna Kirkness, who was the director of the First Nations House of Learning at the University of British Columbia. The quotation appeared as the epigraph to a chapter in Celia Haig-Brown's *Resistance and Renewal: Surviving the Indian Residential School*: "Every time I hear a white person talking about Indians, I get knots in my stomach."[61] Although the book is not so much "about Indians" as it is about white racism and denial, I knew there were blind spots and pitfalls I'd confront, and strong reactions from both Indigenous and non-Indigenous readers who hold to the notion that outsiders have no business talking about such issues. There are plenty of reasons for reacting negatively to the appropriation of stories and artefacts or what might be called the Grey

175

Owl syndrome—assuming Indigenous dress, stories, and songs as a non-Indigenous person. So it's not surprising to find Patricia Monture-Angus, in *Thunder in My Soul: A Mohawk Woman Speaks*, insisting that mainstream scholars and writers cannot "fully understand aboriginal culture as they can never live the life of an Aboriginal person."[62] While I agree with her statement, it also occurs to me that none of us can ever fully understand even the life we or our closest friends and family members live; and that, at times, others can recognize things about us and our condition to which we are completely blind.

After reading Verna Kirkness's challenging comment, I shared my hesitation and uncertainty with Joanie Morris. Her response surprised me.

"Hey, Gary," she laughed, "no one has listened to us for the last two hundred years, so why don't you get off your butt and be the first?"

It was not true, of course, and Joanie knew this, but her comment was an acknowledgement that we all have valuable insights to share about each other's cultures and predicaments. As Wallace Stevens puts it in his famous poem, there are thirteen ways of looking at a blackbird from which a more informed fourteenth impression might emerge. I have come to believe there are no boundaries to the human imagination, and since language is a transforming medium that can, at best, present an altered or different reality from the one we experience through the senses or the intellect, it seems to me that all written versions of a subject, whether penned from inside or outside cultural or ethnic boundaries, are provisional—approximate and mediated visions. I share the view of Alan Cairns, in "First Nations and the Canadian State," the 2002 Kenneth MacGregor Lecture delivered at Queen's University, that, although "Aboriginal scholars bring to this subject an existential empathy that non-Aboriginal scholars cannot command,"[63] the insights of insiders and outsiders can be complementary, knots in the stomach notwithstanding. Those insights, however, should be offered with humility and respect.

The other comment that came my way, from a friend of my wife who knows the terrain much better than I do, was, "I hope Gary has a good support network." I took this to mean that no two Indigenous communities have the same values and challenges and that both Indigenous and non-Indigenous communities have strong opinions about what is proper in terms not only of research activities, but also of what can and cannot be discussed. For example, what are the implications of revealing the dysfunctions and speaking publicly about rogues and bad apples within the Indigenous community? We do this quite readily about non-Indigenous rogues. Writers who have not bothered to consider these questions are likely to end up alienating both communities.

Heather Robertson's *Reservations Are for Indians*—published just a year after Harold Cardinal's *The Unjust Society*—is an important and controversial book. Important because it paints a frank and disturbing portrait of dysfunction and powerlessness in a number of Indigenous communities, and controversial because it traces these problems back to the greed, lies, and bad faith that permeated the treaty process, which Roberston says constituted a blueprint for apartheid.[64] It's a difficult book to read in 2017 because it's not constrained by notions of what's politically correct to say about Indigenous people and because a number of her major concerns about the betrayal of Indigenous rights in the treaty process have in the forty-six intervening years been addressed and thankfully overturned by the Supreme Court.

Robertson offers a detailed account of life in the Norway House Cree Nation, where unemployed men made extra work for themselves by hauling water home in small containers, when two trips with larger buckets instead of six with the small ones would have done the trick, and where the hours spent gossiping and milling around the Bay store had morphed in the minds of participants from a simple means of killing time into something resembling a vital communications network. I was particularly interested in Robertson's description and assessment of the health-care process, which seems to have been one of the few justifications for the Norway House's existence. She calls sickness a "primary industry" and insists that it

> is habit-forming . . . The hospital works frantically at curing and preventing illness, but the harder it tries, the more passive and sick the people become. The hospital thus creates its own patients, along the lines of a capitalist enterprise. Indian and white attitudes work towards one end—to perpetuate the present arrangement.[65]

While hospital staff appeared frustrated at their inability to overcome the medical impasse, Robertson suggests that the recipients of care were equally frustrated. Asking herself why this was happening, she comes to the conclusion that "Indian Affairs makes Indians out of people."[66] The racist ideology declares that these people are helpless children in need of "civilizing" and that we settlers, perhaps as an antidote to white guilt, need to see ourselves as saviours or as healers. She explains in painstaking detail how this process was at work during the signing of the treaties:

> [The treaties were] actually deeds of sale by which the Indians ceded their land to the government. By calling them treaties, the government led the Indians to believe that they were being treated as independent. Actually, behind all the high-flown language of the documents, the government was taking the position that the Indians were not really an independent political group, and by signing the treaties, the Indians unintentionally acknowledged that they were subjects.[67]

What the Indigenous signatories thought were rights were actually restrictions:

> So the British government—and later the Canadian government —created an identity, the status of Indian, and embodied it in the treaties. By signing the treaty, the Indian accepted the position in society and the personality which the British imagined for him. He became a figment of the Anglo-Saxon imagination. He is at least in his official, legal and public self, an artificial creation. The Anglo-Saxon Canadian invented the Indian.[68]

And, of course, the Indian Act of 1880 (Section 12) confirmed this fact by stating, "The term person means an individual other than an Indian."[69]

In describing the Indians as state-created, Robertson sees their poverty as "built in, inescapable."[70] They were land-lease and land-locked peasants at the whim of their landlord, Indian Affairs, and without a citizen's rights to equal land ownership, education, access to health services, freedom of movement, or the right to vote. Even the residential schools maintained the Indigenous person's status as zero, becoming "contagion centres."[71]

In a study from 1941 to 1950 of health conditions amongst the Indigenous peoples in northern Manitoba, Dr. Frederick Tisdall concludes, "'In trying to find out what was at the bottom of this situation we studied the food which the Indians had. We found, according to our present day standards, the Indians received a diet which could not possibly result in good health.'" Robertson also quotes a longer passage where Tisdall describes rotten teeth, repeated pregnancies, anaemia, emaciation, deformity, and other symptoms as "almost universal," and concludes that "[Indians] are not fundamentally indolent and with a lack of initiative. They are sick."[72]

As Robertson suggests, alongside the social segregation came this new segregation by disease. While this is an interesting and important acknowledgement on the part of Tisdall and his colleagues, I'm not comfortable with Robertson's assumptions and conclusions about what she calls "chronic illness and debility" amongst Indigenous peoples: "The diseases are also mainly psychosomatic and sociosomatic. Through his illnesses the Indian stays in touch with Canadian society. As a patient he is important, a problem, so the advantages of disease operate to keep the Indians sick. If they became healthy they might be expelled from the hospital and left to fend on their own in an alien world."[73] This no longer jibes with what we know about the efforts made by Inuit and others to avoid white medicine by hiding or fleeing into the bush, rather than being hijacked and sent south to the sanatoria. Nor does it explain the fear and suspicion so many Indigenous people have of the health-care system, strong enough to make them avoid diagnosis at any cost.

The latter portion of Robertson's book attempts to provide an explanation for the violence, alcoholism, and self-destruction amongst Indigenous peoples. In the case of Lorna, a Métis teenager who was struck and killed at night by an Indigenous drunk driver, Robertson links her death with the fact that she was a rootless orphan, a foster child, and a reluctant former student, whose defiance of the Sisters in her residential school constituted "guerrilla tactics,"[74] an act of civil disobedience in her war against oppression. The suggestion here, and in the example that follows in *Reservations Are for Indians*, is that many such deaths were de facto suicides, since lack of caution and self-care are indicators of extreme depression. A similar argument is mounted to explain alcoholism and what she calls the public spectacle of the Indigenous "drink-in":

Indians have perfectly logical and understandable reason to drink. There is no need to look for disguised aggression as a motive. Any group that is chronically poor, dependent, unemployed, badly educated, and segregated will suffer the tensions and despair that lead to alcoholism. Certainly, Indians in western and northern Canada suffer from all these handicaps. They suffer also from the destruction of their old way of life by contemporary technology, from government restrictions and controls, from the scorn and opprobrium of white Canadians.[75]

As the truth about residential schools had not yet been revealed, Robertson could not have known about the trauma, actual and intergenerational, resulting from physical, emotional, sexual, and cultural abuse. Had she known this, she might have spoken differently about illness. Billie Allan and Janet Smylie, in *First Nations, Second Class Treatment*, give this matter a more contemporary perspective:

> Pointing to the growing body of research in the US and Australia that identifies racism as a chronic stressor implicated in the health of African Americans and Indigenous Australians, the researchers argue for increased research attention to examining the contributions of racism to the persistent health disparities experienced by Indigenous peoples in Canada.[76]

However, I take Robertson's example to be a candid and honest effort, at the time, to describe unsavoury conditions and then trace their causes to unjust and racist decisions put in place by colonial and Canadian lawmakers. Sadly, much of the dysfunction she described happening decades ago that makes glue-sniffing, alcoholism, criminal offences, and the resulting epidemic of early deaths, suicides, and incarceration so tragically common has still not been addressed by our society.

"You must remember that our hearts and brains are like paper; we never forget."

—CHIEF OGICHIDAA,
at the signing of treaties on October 3, 1873

Just Listen

"The problem I have with white people," Joanie Morris has told me more than once, a note of exasperation in her voice, "is that they don't listen."

Apparently, I haven't been paying close enough attention. Either I have been overwhelmed by the information coming my way or a little too concerned with interjecting my own two cents' worth. Or does it have something to do with my placing less value on the spoken word than on the written record? This would be a sorry admission to have to make for someone who has spent a lifetime trying to write poems that nest in the ear and the last three and a half years listening to intimate experiences shared with me by Elders.

The issue of oral history's place in the official archival record of a country, and the value to be placed upon it as evidence, is addressed in an essay by Leslie McCartney called "Respecting First Nations Oral Histories: Copyright Complexities and Archiving Aboriginal Stories." In McCartney's view, "oral forms of history are not given the same protection and respect as literary works under the *Copyright Act.*"[77] With a legal and archival background, and having served as executive director of the Gwich'in Social and Cultural Institute (GSCI) in the Northwest Territories, McCartney is in a good position to discuss this issue and its ramifications.

She approaches the matter anecdotally, considering the official written accounts and literary versions of the Albert Johnson story and the importance placed upon them as against the Gwich'in oral accounts that tend to be overlooked, but which contain important cultural information. I won't try to reconstruct her essay, but I mention it here to acknowledge the importance of the issue. If, as she insists, "all stories are constructed by reading the past selectively,"[78] then oral history ought not to be ignored or marginalized.

I recall Barry Broadfoot's *Ten Lost Years* and *Six War Years*, two books of oral history interviews that owed much to the great Studs Turkel and provided moving, personal accounts of living through those tumultuous times that could not be found in the official history texts. They were galvanizing for me in a way that no history text on the subjects had been, in part because of the intimacy, the specific detail, and the sense of a survivor's authentic voice. They felt less constructed than most written accounts, though I could imagine that much of their power had come from the stories having been refined in the retelling, or re-remembering, over a lifetime. The oral accounts from the Great Depression may have been constructed through the lenses of class or ideology and the war stories through the lenses of class and rank, but they seemed, nevertheless, to float freely in the books, distinct and unfettered by an overriding narrative, the relevance to what I am struggling to do here duly noted.

For those who still feel oral history is less reliable than the written stuff, here's a reminder that socially constructed narratives of the written variety also require considerable scrutiny and analysis. While I was doing my research, my friend Jim Anderson, an antiquarian bookseller and budding writer in Winnipeg, sent me about twenty photocopied pages from *Forty-four Years with the Northern Crees* [sic], published in 1942 by Christian missionary S.D. Gaudin. Jim felt the book had some revealing passages about attitudes to residential schools and Indigenous health. The introduction, by fellow missionary Kenneth J. Beaton, sets a rather jarring tone for today's reader as it broaches the subject of religious memoirs:

> Adventure, romance, courage and consecration are to be found at every turn, and yet many of the greatest stories have never been recorded. Our literature describing the work which turned roving nomad tribes, ignorant, illiterate, dirty and disease-ridden into intelligent Christian communities is very meagre.[79]

Just as I'm thinking "not meagre enough," Beaton, without an ounce of awareness that residential schools were still plying their grizzly trade, lists the apparent rewards: "The great gifts of a written language, of vocational education, of training in personal hygiene and public health and the emergence of Indian leadership in a few generations, make a thrilling and encouraging record."

The actual memoir is more culturally sensitive than this appalling introduction, providing a few examples of the Gaudins' care and generosity. Yet, in a paragraph that describes Gaudin leaving his wife and children with friends in Moose Jaw in order to deliver eight Indigenous children to a school in Red Deer, after the Brandon Residential School has refused to accept them because they're non-treaty, the tragic outcome of the journey is offered with no comment whatsoever on the justice, policies, or conditions of residential schools: "In the course of two or three years five of those apparently healthy children had died from Tuberculosis."[80]

Later, in a mix-up over appointments that sends the Gaudins to new work in Cross Lake instead of Norway House, four Indigenous children entrusted to their keeping don't fare too well: "again there was disaster for two were in their graves before Christmas" and a third saved only by the exceptional interventions of Mrs. Gaudin.[81] While it's clear that he cares about these losses, Gaudin does not, even at the supposedly wise age of eighty-one when the book was published, openly question the logic of a school system that ends up killing five out of eight and two out of four children. That's a combined average of 56.5 per cent—a record consistent with Dr. Peter Bryce's results in 1907, when his examination of the Indian residential schools in the prairies reported deaths in the 40 to 60 per cent range.

There are many ways to consider the pros and cons of oral history and how these matters affect our understanding of Indigenous health. Velvet Maud, a Manitoba Métis woman, with whom I exchanged emails, considers several of them in her master's thesis in Native Studies at the University of Saskatchewan, titled "Understanding Narratives of Illness and Contagion as a Strategy to Prevent Tuberculosis among Métis in Southern Manitoba." Her thesis is especially useful in terms of the historical background of TB and its various treatments. I had not known, for example, that lobectomy refers to the removal of a part of a lung, whereas pneumonectomy refers to its full removal; or that the latter resulted in an average 40 per cent cure, 40 per cent death, and 20 per cent neither. Much of her information is drawn from former patients of Ninette Sanatorium, the first in Manitoba, opened in 1910 at Pelican Lake. Even more importantly, I learned that streptomycin, a cure for TB invented by Dr. Selman Waksman in the US, was available as early as 1944, but could only be accessed by those with money; the drug would not be freely available in Manitoba until 1953.[82]

Maud makes a strong case for studying the oral narratives and stigmas surrounding tuberculosis because so many of them indicate that misconceptions about the disease and how it spread had resulted in unnecessary infections and deaths. Her own grandmother, for example, who tried to keep her tuberculosis a secret, thought she had contracted the disease from a cook who spat in her soup. As Maud explained to me in an email:

> I know exactly how difficult it is to get people to open up and tell you their stories. I did interviews for my MA, and I found people were more than willing to talk to me, until I mentioned I was doing research and then most slammed the door on me and I totally understand why. My grandmother, a Métis woman, spent about 6 years in sanatoriums (Ninette, St. Boniface both in MB & Pearson Hospital in Vancouver) and did not have a pleasant experience at any of the locations. She seldom spoke of her time at the TB sanatorium, but the odd time she would let something out, like being pressured to have an abortion in 1947 for the sake of her health and refusing (she had already done one stint at Ninette). The doctors were right and she had to be re-admitted. The next time she became pregnant, in 1950, she took the doctor's advice, fearing the TB would become active again. I do not think my grandma was involved with any experiments or sexually or physically abused but her time in the hospital did affect her mentally, spiritually, and emotionally until the day she died and it did impact at least three generations of my family.

184

As Maud suggests in another email, oral family narratives of disease are not always so far off the mark:

> I know another woman whose grandfather was sent to the sanatorium without ever having TB. The doctor in the community figured he had too

many children so to keep him from reproducing he admitted him to the sanatorium. I do not understand the logic behind this but as his grand-daughter said, it was a method to keep down the half-breed population.

While we don't know whether this was a case of forced absence as a means of contraception or if the intention was to administer an involuntary vasectomy while the grandfather was in the hospital, both possibilities are equally disturbing.

Although her own research depends predominantly on the documentary record, Maureen Lux generously recommended that I read Julie Cruikshank's essay, "Oral Tradition and Oral History: Reviewing Some Issues," where the debate over the relative merits of oral and written history is put simply:

> This debate is as much about epistemology as about authorship. Indigenous people who grow up in oral tradition frequently suggest that their narratives are better understood by absorbing the successive personal messages revealed to listeners in repeated tellings than by trying to analyse and publicly explain their meanings. This contrasts with a scholarly approach which encourages close scrutiny of texts and which contends that by openly addressing conflicting interpretations, we may illuminate subtle meanings and enrich our understanding. The challenge, then, is to acknowledge this dilemma without dismissing it as insoluble, to respect both the legitimate claims of First Nations to tell their own stories and the moral and scholarly obligations to write culturally grounded histories that can help us learn from the past.[83]

Cruikshank goes on to outline various opinions and approaches to oral history, but shares the view that oral and written histories are mediated, their materials shaped and interpreted, with elements both subjective and objective.[84] If written history has a limited lifespan (say, one or two decades), the reliability of oral histories should hardly be an issue. Her brief account of David Cohen's experience in Uganda, where powerful clans managed to record their oral histories, thereby gaining added authority over those who did not have the resources to do the same, raises interesting questions in my mind about the relative merits of the oral accounts of Indigenous–settler relations provided by those who have left behind their traditional beliefs and adopted the conqueror's religion. Are their oral histories any less reliable as a result? Will their interpretation of the violent, or even gradual, overthrowing of traditional ways be different? Or, when individual and collective memories coincide, is this reason enough to privilege them?

Many questions remain unanswered. However, one of the main values of oral history, in my mind, is that it can challenge or destabilize the written narrative of the victors who, as we know, always get to write the official, if not always the most reliable, version of events.

Issues of orality and listening remind me of Margaret Atwood's "Two-Headed Poems," in which she describes the French-English conflicts in Canada as "a duet with two deaf singers."[85] Unfortunately, time spent on that important French–English duet has left a lot of Canadians tone deaf and indifferent to the rich choir of voices and concerns of Canada's Indigenous peoples. Hugh Brody, author of *Maps and Dreams* and one of the most articulate advocates for Indigenous rights in Canada's north, offers this useful reminder for those of us with ears: "Listening is difficult; hearing even more so."[86]

A notable exception to Canadian deafness or indifference is Larry Frolick, whose recent work, *Crow Never Dies: Life on the Great Hunt*, exemplifies the kind of listening and close attention needed if we are to understand our Indigenous brothers and sisters. Frolick invites the reader on a moving and instructive journey into life in the north as it is still lived by many of its Gwich'in inhabitants, a hard life that requires constant attention and stamina to survive the rigours of the hunt and the austere climate in challenging terrain. Frolick takes the time to enter into these lives and ways, spending long periods hunting, listening, and speculating about what he has experienced, never assuming he knows it all, and always deferring to the superior wisdom of his teachers on the land who see, understand, and remember so much more than he, as guest and visitor, can comprehend. He even refers to himself in the text on occasion as "the writer," thereby undercutting his own authority as first-person narrator, a reminder to himself and readers that he is only an observer of the complicated web of practice, story, and memory that keeps the Indigenous northerner and his or her culture alive, adapting to the constant changes, including the seasons, the land, the migration of animals, and the intrusion of settlers.

The earlier chapters of Frolick's book move slowly, which is appropriate for a non-fiction work that is not driven by plot or a specific journey, but rather by the wisdom to be derived from a variety of chance meetings. However, the pace picks up as the book progresses, the second half packed with animal encounters (including a sly, determined grizzly that swims silently, unnoticed and ever closer to the stern of Frolick's boat), hunting lore, and arduous journeys in an unrelenting but striking land.

The self-deprecating humour—Frolick's own fears, anxiety, and ignorance set against the wisdom and seeming nonchalance of his guides or companions—gives the book an added dimension, not only endearing us to the narrator, but also inviting us to share his wonder and willingness to ponder. The result is that we begin to understand and hold in awe a way of life that we might have once dismissed as primitive, passé, or inferior but which, in fact, is shown to be subtle, complicated, and heroic in comparison to the technology-laden and overly protected world of privilege many of us inhabit.

I am in awe of Frolick's wisdom and humility as an interpreter of Gwich'in and northern ways. Equally admirable is his ability to adapt the style of narrating to the material at hand, by which I mean he is prepared to leave jargon and the high style of academic writing behind, thus lessening the contrast between the wise, earthy orality of his hosts and the often pompous and convoluted jargon of the scholar. While he avoids the worst trappings of scholarly writing, he manages with great panache to transmit huge amounts of information with seeming effortlessness, and in a style at times unobtrusively poetic.

An intriguing perspective on written and oral cultures was provided many years ago by cultural anthropologist Claude Levi-Strauss, who suggested that "the primary function of writing, as a means of communication, is to facilitate the enslavement of other human beings."[87] It's a bold statement, but we know something about the power and authority invested in written language from current challenges to the so-called contracts and treaties by which imperial nations and vested interests justified the theft of Indigenous lands. And we know the power of holy books, scriptures, and papal nuncios in controlling people's lives.

In *A Long and Terrible Shadow: White Values, Native Rights in the Americas since 1492*, Justice Thomas Berger explores the battle government lawyers fought to deny Indigenous title in Canada, focussing on the long struggle of the Nisga'a for recognition in British Columbia. What it boiled down to is quite simple, Berger says: "They could not accept that people without a written language can, nevertheless, have an elaborate legal system of their own."[88] After several defeats in court, however, Indigenous title was finally acknowledged by Justice Emmett Hall, who declared, "What emerges from the . . . evidence is that the [Nisga'a] in fact are and were from time immemorial a distinctive cultural entity with concepts of ownership indigenous to their culture and capable of articulation under common law."[89]

I began this chapter with a quotation by Chief Ogichidaa, so it's fitting to end with a recent statement by his successors on the current state of affairs, which touches upon the issues of memory and the importance of listening. In the "Submission to the Ipperwash Inquiry," the Grand Council of Treaty #3 makes strong claims for the Anishinaabe people as a sovereign nation, with rights to hunt and fish and be consulted about development projects on their traditional lands. The Council points out that consultation about land claims and Indigenous rights, if the issue comes up at all, is always an "afterthought," and that historical mistrust exists as a result of racism, not only at the government level, but also in the justice system, manifested in undue incarceration, police brutality, and failure to act in cases of the beatings and homicides of Indigenous people at the hands of white youth, citing the case of the KIB (Kenora Indian Bashers), whose members act with complete impunity in the area. The report concludes:

> Racism is alive and thriving in the Treaty #3 area. Why, because the governments continue to condone such attitudes and behaviours of its own institutions' personnel by doing nothing about the problem of racism. Just recently, the *Winnipeg Free Press* ran a story of how the mayors and town leaders of Kenora, Fort Frances, and Rainy River area reported that they felt ignored by southern Ontario and talked about becoming part of Manitoba. If the white leaders feel ignored by their own governments, how can the First Nation people expect to be heard?[90]

The Council asks how their people can be expected to move forward under such conditions, but somehow manages to move beyond justifiable rage and once again extend the hand of sharing and partnership:

> It is one thing to forgive and move forward but when unnecessary deaths of our people continue to happen in this day and age, there is never any moving forward, just the recurring memories of seeing our parents humiliated and our sense of helplessness as children of how society views the "original people of this land." But, we are the survivors of our nation, and while we still have many struggles to overcome, we are prepared to work together with you to make the changes that are necessary so we can all live together in peace and harmony.[91]

twenty-seven

Who Wrote the Menu?

We're meeting in a restaurant called The Salisbury House at the intersection of Stafford Street and Pembina Highway in Winnipeg, a place that, like the two of us, has seen better days but continues to thrive. I am squinting through a pair of five-year-old glasses, my prescription ones having broken the night before leaving home on this trip. And Ted Fontaine is using a walker and taking his time getting into the booth. The Salisbury survived different owners until being taken over in 2006 by a group of investors that includes Burton Cummings, lead singer of The Guess Who. Though neither upscale nor flashy, it's still acknowledged by Winnipeggers to serve the best burgers in town, known locally as "nips."

Having just nipped into town, I'm delighted with the opportunity to meet this celebrated author and Elder, a member and former chief of the Sagkeeng Ojibway First Nation. Theodore Fontaine is the author of *Broken Circle*, a memoir of his years spent in the Fort Alexander Indian Residential School ninety miles north of Winnipeg. In this touching account, he points a finger at some of the problems his people faced dealing with the legacy of residential schools, including "an overabundance of unhealthy fats, starchy food, carbohydrates, sugar, and salt"[92] endured by the unfortunate students and Indigenous staff, while the smells of tastier, healthier meals wafted from the faculty dining area. The long-term effects of persistent hunger and bad diet in the schools were often reinforced later at home.

Many diseases and other health problems First Nations suffer today, Ted explains,

> stem from intergenerational attitudes and what survivors inadvertently pass on to their children, sometimes with the misguided intent to make life better and less painful for them. Parental guilt over losing children to residential schools resulted in widespread resolve by parents to compensate for not fighting enough to keep us home. When we went home in the summers, we'd be showered with practically anything we wanted if it could be afforded, including a lot of candy, pop and other unhealthy snacks.

Hunger is certainly a major theme surfacing in many of my interviews with Elders, not just the shortage of food and an inadequate diet in residential schools, but also extreme malnutrition in the wider community, where white encroachment and new restrictions on fishing, hunting, and the gathering of wild crops reduced the independence and self-sufficiency of Indigenous peoples. James Daschuk has written powerfully on this subject in *Clearing the Plains*. He documents how the tribes, despite the promises of Treaty 6, were deliberately starved to make way for the railway and settlement, and how this policy was not just something set in motion by Indian agents and corrupt suppliers, but official government policy endorsed by Prime Minister John A. Macdonald. In an interview with musician and New Democrat MP Charlie Angus, Daschuk talks about Treaty 6, in which the government clearly committed itself to famine and pestilence relief but within a couple of years broke its promises. When interviewer Angus expresses his shock at what he calls the "bureaucratization of misery," Daschuk quotes Macdonald's self-congratulatory boast to parliament that he is deliberately keeping the Indians on the verge of "actual starvation."[93] The rationale was simple. Outright massacre was no longer politically acceptable, but keeping the Indians so hungry that their immune systems were compromised, leaving them harmless and susceptible to tuberculosis and other deadly diseases, was considered wise policy. Thus, the Indigenous people of the Great Plains, independent, fed on a diet of buffalo, and once described as the tallest and proudest of warriors, were brought to their knees.

Daschuk, responding in the *Globe and Mail* to Ian Mosby's article on nutritional experiments on Indigenous children, reminds us that there is nothing new in the story of drug and medical experiments, as the politics of starvation was used to clear the prairies. His conclusion is a reminder of what needs to be acknowledged if we are to move ahead:

> As the skeletons in our collective closet are exposed to the light, through the work of Dr. Mosby and others, perhaps we will come to understand the uncomfortable truths that modern Canada is founded upon—ethnic cleansing and genocide—and push our leaders and ourselves to make a nation we can be proud to call home.[94]

Maureen Lux has also written extensively on Indigenous health in the prairies. In *Medicine That Walks*, she considers hunger and poverty to be the main cause of the ill health and near decimation of Canada's Indigenous peoples. But her thoughts on medicine are equally important and engaging. While traditional medicines would have helped stave off disease in normal circumstances—the Blackfoot had numerous treatments for skin diseases and even more for respiratory diseases—Lux says that at least 50 per cent of them died from smallpox in 1837–38, and a similar plague inflicted severe losses on the Assiniboine.[95] Traditional cures would have helped had the population been well fed and rooted in the home place where they could gather medicines. Plains Indigenous people survived these and other losses, but the one they could not survive was the loss of the buffalo, millions of which were slaughtered by hunters and traders in the 1870s. This fact alone drove the two groups mentioned, along with the Cree and Saultaux and other tribes and nations, to enter into treaty talks, in which medicine chests, an annual financial pittance, and ample provisions were promised. In addition to her conviction that "starvation at Fort Walsh was a cynical and deliberate plan to press to the government advantage and force the Cree from the area to allow the government a free hand in developing the prairies,"[96] Lux concludes that the entire treaty process was criminally flawed:

Aboriginal people had been promised just eight years earlier that by "taking the Queen's hand" in treaty, they would have a future. Instead, they were caught in a vicious circle of malnutrition, which weakens the immune system, and infection. Nearly any endemic illness can become epidemic during famine—especially typhus, smallpox, dysentery, tuberculosis, influenza, and pneumonia. This synergism between common infections and malnutrition accounted for the increased mortality and morbidity.[97]

Having made her point so powerfully, with pages of statistics to back it up, she moves on to the issue of medicine and healing, spending many pages talking about traditional medical practices, including botanical cures and midwifery.

It should be apparent from what I've written so far that the single most important threats to Indigenous health in the nineteenth and twentieth centuries were displacement, hunger, and residential schools, where disease was the unavoidable byproduct of emotional, physical, and sexual abuse. Lux has no doubt about the unholy marriage between early religious schools and segregated hospitals. "The connection was intimate by design," she writes. "Children who became ill in school would not have to be sent home and could remain on the school rolls."[98] A similar situation would prevail between the residential schools and segregated Indian hospitals in the twentieth century, in cahoots not only in the maintaining of numbers and funding, but also in providing guinea pigs for drug and surgical experiments and electric shock treatment. In terms of serious medical care, Lux argues, treaty promises had long since been forgotten or ignored by a government whose "policy was borne of parsimony."[99] This policy, which included sporadic or non-existent doctor's visits as well as flawed and inadequate vaccines, resulted in immense suffering and huge numbers of unnecessary deaths. If all this seems like genocide in the making, conditions were in place for the next major killer, tuberculosis.

By 1932, BCG vaccines, which had shown some effectiveness in reducing the death rate and controlling the spread of tuberculosis, were still being debated in Canada. As Lux argues, "American and Canadian policies toward Native people's health were driven by the same goals—assimilation and the protection of non-Natives," the prime concern being "how to confine the disease to the reserves."[100] In the 1940s and 1950s, three drugs—streptomycin, para-aminosalicylic acid, and isonicotinic acid hydrazide—became available and proved to be effective in treating tuberculosis. It would seem, then, that the emphasis on excessive rest and surgical intervention would have ceased immediately, but this was not the case. A captive audience of guinea pigs would not be easily surrendered, as we can see from the medical and nutritional experiments of the 1950s and early 1960s and the forced sterilizations that continued apace.

This is where the conclusions of Daschuk, Lux, and Fontaine agree: all things considered, poverty, displacement, abuse, broken promises, residential schools, and other forms of ethnic cleansing have continued to be the main causes of illness and premature death amongst First Nations, Métis, and Inuit peoples in Canada. And the combination surely explains the current sad spectacle of hardship, unemployment, alcoholism, dysfunction, and suicide amongst Indigenous populations.

As our luncheon continues, I learn that there's hardly an institution in Manitoba to which Ted Fontaine has not contributed his skills and wisdom, from health, finance, employment, and governance issues to conflict resolution. His record of achievements is all the more remarkable given the negative reinforcement he received in residential school, where "the nuns and priests had taught us that we could not ever have the jobs of the bosses. My confidence plummeted as I was exposed to more and more of these superior attitudes."[101] He has no difficulty, either in his memoir or in discussion, identifying racism and colonialism as the poisons that profoundly impacted so many of his generation.

"Most residential school survivors avoid direct eye contact. The blame that's mostly turned inward has caused shame." He looks me in the eye as our discussion comes to an end, and I'm reminded of his comment in *Broken Circle*: "Although genocide has often been denied in Canada, history shows that soon after the appearance of Columbus in the Americas around 1500, the practice of hunting and killing Indian people began."[102]

While Ted and I discuss shame, hunger, and other serious matters, we're munching on a couple of Winnipeg's best burgers, or nips, looking anything but starved or malnourished. As he prepares to leave, I look around the restaurant noting the appropriateness of the musical instruments on the walls, some of them doubtless selected or donated by co-owner Burton Cummings, who's only seven years younger than I am. All we need now, to make the moment even more resonant, are the refrains of a couple of his hit tunes, say, "Share the Land" and "No Time."

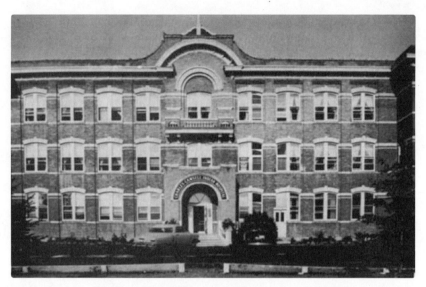

↑ Charles Camsell Indian Hospital, Edmonton, Alberta. 'HON. BROOKE CLAXTON' N.D., CA. NOVEMBER 1945, PT I, FILE 800-I-D479, VOL. 2592, RG29, LIBRARY AND ARCHIVES CANADA

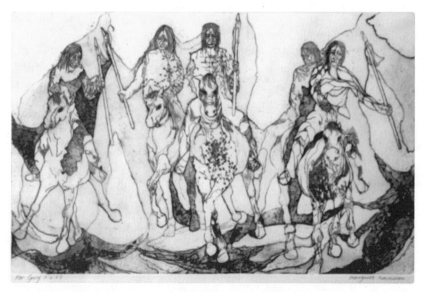

↑ *Les Cavaliers Fantômes*, an etching by Margaret Nashchen.

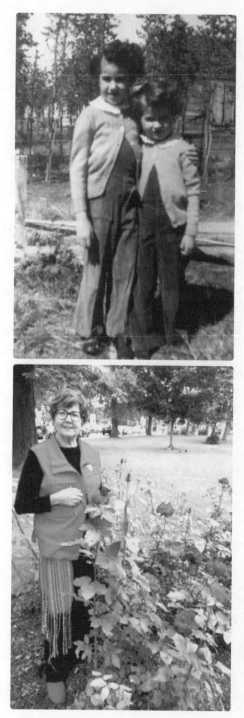

← Marilyn Murray-Allison with little
sister Pam. MARILYN MURRAY-ALLISON
COLLECTION

← Marilyn Murray-Allison at home
in Victoria. COURTESY SISTER PAM

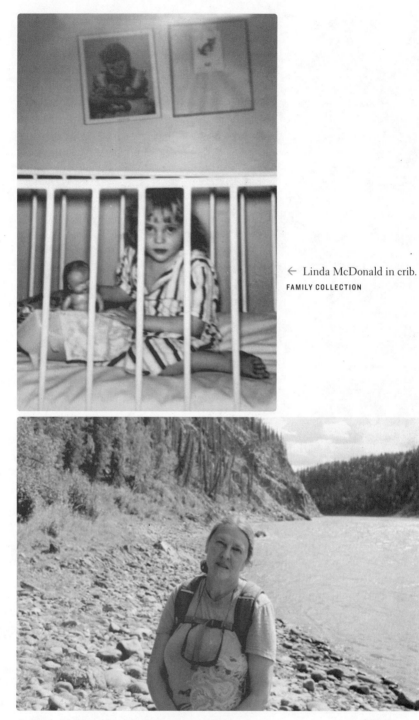

← Linda McDonald in crib.

↑ Linda McDonald in Liard Canyon. LESLIE MAIN JOHNSON

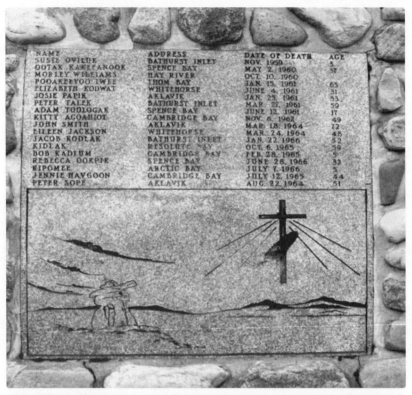

NAME	ADDRESS	DATE OF DEATH	AGE
SUSIE OVILUK	BATHURST INLET	NOV. 1959	5
OOTAK KAKFANOOK	SPENCE BAY	MAY 2, 1960	37
MORLEY WILLIAMS	HAY RIVER	OCT. 10, 1960	
POOAKEEYOO IWEE	THOM BAY	JAN. 15, 1961	65
ELIZABETH KODWAT	WHITEHORSE	JUNE 4, 1961	31
JOSIE PAPIK	AKLAVIK	JAN. 25, 1961	53
PETER TALEK	BATHURST INLET	MAR. 21, 1961	59
ADAM TOOLOGAK	SPENCE BAY	JUNE 12, 1961	17
KITTY AGOAHIOT	CAMBRIDGE BAY	NOV. 6, 1962	49
JOHN SMITH	AKLAVIK	MAR. 18, 1964	72
EILEEN JACKSON	WHITEHORSE	MAR. 24, 1964	48
JACOB KODLAK	BATHURST INLET	JAN. 22, 1966	52
KIDLAK	RESOLUTE BAY	OCT. 4, 1965	39
BOB RADIUM	CAMBRIDGE BAY	FEB. 28, 1965	5
REBECCA OOKPIK	SPENCE BAY	JUNE 28, 1966	32
KIPOMEE	ARCTIC BAY	JULY 1, 1966	5
JENNIE HAVGOON	CAMBRIDGE BAY	JULY 12, 1965	44
PETER SOPE	AKLAVIK	AUG. 22, 1964	51

↑ Memorial for Camsell dead. GARY GEDDES

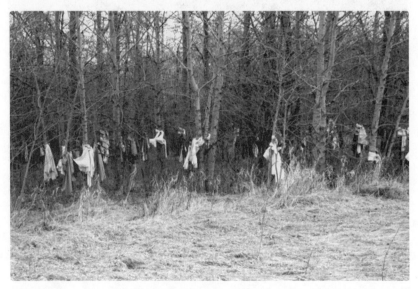

↑ Prayer flags at Poundmaker's Lodge Treatment Centre. GARY GEDDES

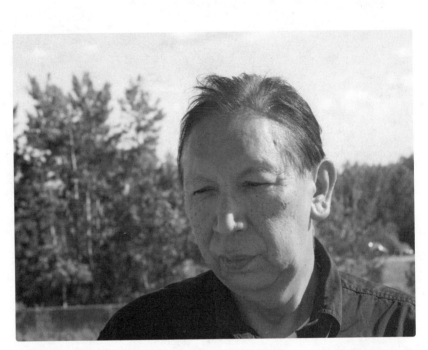

↑ Clifford Cardinal. GARY GEDDES

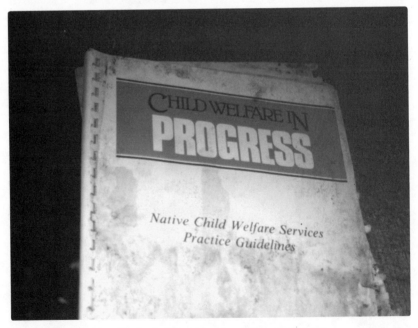

↑ Child Welfare pamphlet in abandoned nursing station. GARY GEDDES

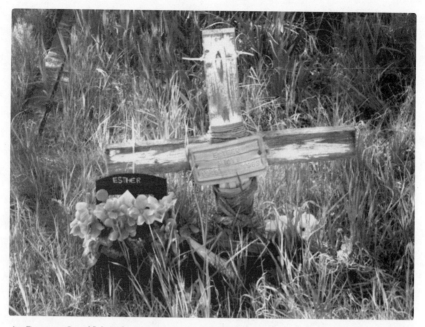

↑ Grave at Goodfish Lake cemetery. **GARY GEDDES**

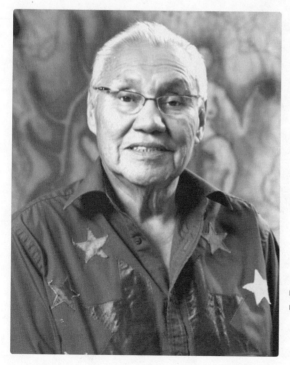

← Noel Starblanket.
PHOTOGRAPHY DEPT.,
UNIVERSITY OF REGINA

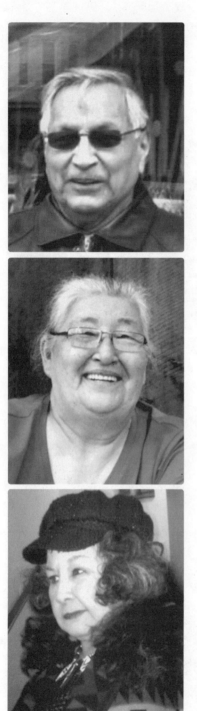

← Bill Asikinack. ANONYMOUS FRIEND

← Lorraine Yuzicapi. HOLLY RAE YUZICAPI

← Eleanor James-Robertson. JULIAN ROBERTSON

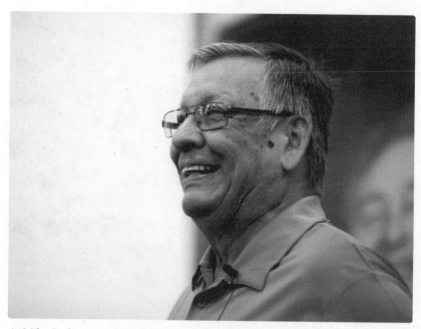

↑ Mike Cachagee. **ALGOMA UNIVERSITY**

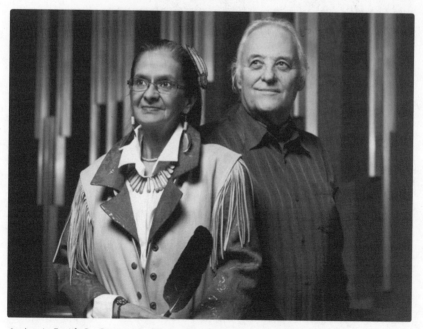

↑ Annie Smith St. Georges and Robert St. Georges. **NATIONAL ARTS CENTRE**

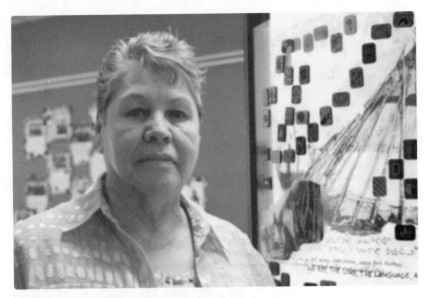

↑ Shirley Horn. SHIRLEY HORN COLLECTION

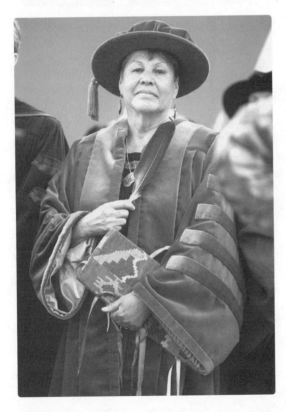

← Chancellor Shirley Horn,
Algoma University.
KENNETH ARMSTRONG

PART THREE

THE LONG
SENTENCE

And the First Shall
Be Last

twenty-eight

Tidbits, the Mush Hole, and Bovine TB

The imposition of artificial provincial and territorial boundaries in Canada divided Indigenous peoples and placed them under different jurisdictions, but it did not stop their movement once the pass system was abolished. However, these boundaries did have a negative effect on access to health care. I have heard numerous stories of patients with tuberculosis and other diseases that required immediate attention languishing in a medical limbo as health institutions and authorities dickered over who had the responsibility and who would pay the bill.

At the moment, I am not only paying the bill but also having a snack with Bill Asikinack at Tim Horton's on Albert Street in the south end of Regina, while his tiny black dog waits for him in a huge black SUV parked outside. Bill graciously accepts my gifts of Virginia Shag tobacco and smoked salmon from the Mad Dog Crab fish shop in Duncan, BC. As we sip our respective drinks—his a medium roast coffee and mine a hot chocolate—he tells me about growing up on Walpole Island in southwestern Ontario, living with his adoptive parents on the reserve, and attending the local day school. Because his grandmother lived between his home and the school, he would sometimes stop in to enjoy her company, stories, and a cup of tea, a prospect that proved more interesting and instructive than what passed for education in the classroom. After Bill missed six days of school—three beyond the allowable limit—the Indian agent arrived and announced that he would be transferred to the residential school and, as punishment, spend grades one to six there, one year for each day of school missed. When I remark that it would be an understatement to call this a gross miscarriage of justice, he refers to the passage in the Indian Act that gives the agent authority to remove children and determine their fate. So, at age six, Bill was declared a criminal and sent off as punishment to the Mush Hole, otherwise known as the Mohawk Institute, in Brantford, Ontario.

Bill's leg began to trouble him towards the end of his time at residential school, with pain and swelling at the knee, but no one paid much attention to the problem, other than sending him to bed. Only when he returned home in June was the problem taken seriously. He started grade seven at the reserve school in September, but by December the leg was worse and the family doctor had diagnosed the problem as tuberculosis of the bone. By January, Bill found himself at the sanatorium in Windsor, Ontario.

The disease—later called osteomyelitis, a bone infection that responds to antibiotics—was treated in those days by debridement, the surgical removal of damaged or necrotic tissue. At the San, Bill explains, he underwent careful monitoring and then some rather brutal surgical interventions that left him lame, his left leg two inches shorter than the right. He pulls up his pant leg to show me the nasty scars where the scraping was done and metal pins were inserted.

Ambient noise is louder than usual at Tim Horton's. I adjust the tape recorder to full volume, hoping Bill's story can be heard above the acoustic tsunami that has engulfed us. He's replying to my question about the cause of his tuberculosis. I've offered what I know about children being deliberately infected at residential schools by being forced to share desks and beds with classmates who had open sores or infected lungs. Many kids already known to be sick were admitted to the residential schools to boost enrolment, thereby prompting an increase in government funding. But Bill has done his research and found a series of letters from Indian Affairs to the residential school administration that point to a different source.

"Milk," he tells me, licking the sticky sugar of Tim's apple fritters from his fingers and thumb. I'm doing the same, having made the wrong choice of snack for both of us. "The cows were contaminated and we got sick from the milk. Official letters to the school principal confirmed this and demanded that all the cows be destroyed." It's not enough that loneliness, stress, and all manner of abuse should undermine the children's immune systems; even the complacent bovines turned out to be complicit.

The accompanying stories about his ward-mates at the sanatorium don't inspire much confidence in the medical professionals, who seem to have been flying by the seat of their pants at best, even in the '50s when antibiotics became available. One tubercular child apparently could not be cured without removing his arm above the elbow. A German-Canadian twin died from TB. Another patient recovered and returned to the reserve, where he became a barber. Bill has lost track of the others, although he remembers some of their names. I ask if he's considered knee replacement procedures, which would at least give him the capacity to lengthen and bend his left leg. He takes another swig of coffee and laughs at the suggestion.

"What, all that time in the hospital at my age? Even with the offer of extending my leg another two inches, I'd rather endure the pain and discomfort."

I have friends who were released from the hospital within days of their knee replacement operation, so I'm wondering if Bill knows this or is responding on the basis of old, unpleasant hospital experiences.

Bill's age is eighty, but in spite of the pain and challenges of his life, he looks about sixty-five. I ask him about anger. Where does it go? How has he handled it, when all around him progress for First Nations, Métis, and Inuit people has been so difficult and so slow? We talk a bit about the Oka crisis. Then he gives me a list of Indigenous success stories, including Cree playwright Tomson Highway, of whom we both have amusing stories, his about Tomson deciding to come out of the closet and being surprised when Bill said, "Why bother, you're just a two-spirit person, something that's totally acceptable to our people." Mine is about Tomson's warning when I picked him up at the airport in Vancouver to do some readings and talks in Bellingham, Washington: "Plan to stop often, Gary. I drink eight glasses of water each morning, so I'll have to pee every ten miles." Then Bill talks about his former students, Perry Bellegarde, the new chief of the Assembly of First Nations, and the great Abenaki filmmaker Alanis Obomsawin, whose *Kanehsatake: 270 Years of Resistance* analyzes and defines the Oka crisis in Quebec.

I acknowledge these successes but wonder about the many who have suffered and not had the strength or the opportunities to rise above their pain. Role models are important, but they don't eliminate personal or collective anger, which is too often turned against the self, the family, and the community. Bill refuses to go down that path.

"Sure, there's plenty to be angry about. Hold on to your anger, but don't let it consume you. Exercise control. Otherwise the anger escalates and consumes you. I was at a special First Nations ceremony once when this subject came up. There was a lot of clamour. We were reminded of the advice of the Old Ones about the need for education: 'Learn the cunning of the white man if you want to succeed in this new world.' That's when a special guest advised us to 'do something positive with your anger.' Can you guess who that was?" When I can't come up with the right answer, Bill provides it: "The famous Piapot Cree singer/songwriter, Buffy Sainte Marie."

The unceded territory of Bkejwanong, "where the waters divide," also known as Walpole Island, which Bill locates easily on the screen of his cell phone, is in the mouth of the St. Clair River in southwestern Ontario, across the water from Michigan. He takes pride in showing me photographs of his family, a nephew receiving an award from a forestry company, a son who is an arborist, and three sisters, two of whom were students at Shingwauk Residential School. Although he's a proud family man and an active community member, my homework suggests that Bill Asikinack has also turned his anger into other major achievements. He completed a BA in social sciences at the University of Western Ontario, as well as Master's in educational administration, and he is registered for the PhD at University of Regina. He was a coordinator of Adult Cultural Programming for ten years before becoming the head of Indigenous Studies at the University of Regina.

A popular and exemplary teacher, "Mr. Bill" writes reviews, articles, and books, including *Explorations into North America*, which was translated into several languages, and *Exploring History*, co-authored with Kate Scarborough. While Bill makes a phone call, I persuade the clerk at Tim's to give me some wet napkins to rinse our sticky hands. Then, ever the teacher, Bill regales me with tidbits (not Timbits) about Indigenous and European history that few know, including the fact that it was not Sir Walter Raleigh who brought tobacco to England from the Americas, although he took the credit; it was his son. And for those who think the Irish invented and then died from the lack of potatoes, he's happy to let them know that the humble vegetable originated in the Americas.

Although dismissing anger as a strategy for change, Bill is no stranger to irony and there's nothing sugar-coated about his assessment of the situation of his people.

"To get back to the Mush Hole for a moment," he says, "we were marched along the street every Sunday to attend services at the Anglican Church nearby and forced to sing as we went."

I'm a step ahead of him for the first and only time.

"'Onward Christian Soldiers'?"

"You got it."

twenty-nine

Poisoned Earth and Deaf Ears_____

"**W**hat, they didn't die? Now what?"
I am listening to the voice of Anishinaabe comedian Ryan McMahon on his radio program *Red Man Laughing*, describing the average Canadian's shock in the not-so-distant past to discover there were still Indians around and that they were not happy campers on tiny postage stamp portions of what they considered their own land. McMahon is interviewing Wab Kinew shortly after the publication of his book *The Reason You Walk*. It's a splendid book and an insightful interview, during which the two men share some very personal feelings about the past and the road ahead for their people and for the rest of Canada.

Kinew begins by insisting that reconciliation is not just a social justice issue but an opportunity for all of us to become better human beings. An issue in the book was his father's controversial decision towards the end of his life to adopt the Archbishop of Winnipeg as his brother. While many saw this as appalling, Wab sees it as a process that helped him and his father mature and reconnect with the core Anishinaabe values of love, kindness, sharing, and respect.

"It's not enough to be right," he says, meaning the right side of history. "You also have to be good."[1]

The alternative is to let anger reduce you to the level of your oppressor, where you perpetuate the legacy of the residential school, segregated hospitals, and other blessings of the colonial system. McMahon agrees that

211

it takes more effort to hold onto anger than to try do something productive with it.

Both McMahon and Kinew come from a beautiful area of lakes and forests around the Manitoba–Ontario border that has been degraded by mining, clear-cutting, and industrial pollution at considerable cost to the health and wellbeing of the original inhabitants. I'm thinking in particular of the horror story of mercury poisoning at Grassy Narrows in the 1970s caused by the Dryden mill, now known as Reed Paper, and its adjoining chemical plant in northwestern Ontario. The mill has come into the news again as a result of a new push to log huge tracts of land, where the resulting run-off is considered likely to increase pollution in local rivers. Protests in the 1970s resulted in national and international attention. The Japanese doctor Masazumi Harada spent considerable time in Canada testing First Nations individuals in Grassy Narrows and Whitedog, the two endangered reserves, convinced they too were suffering from Minamata disease, the toxic scourge that had ravaged lives, causing death and deformities in Japan as a result of mercury released by the Chisson Corporation's plant in Minamata Bay.

Typically, Indigenous protests resulted in denial and empty promises from government and industry. Information from labs in Ottawa—where the fact that cats given large amounts of contaminated fish from the Wabigoon and English Rivers soon developed the neurological damage and erratic behaviour known as the "dance of death" caused by mercury poisoning—was kept under wraps. Closure of the fisheries caused havoc among not only lodge owners, but also Indigenous guides and residents who depended on employment and income from tourism and for whom fish was a traditional food source. Reed Paper was the principal employer around which the city of Dryden had risen. The fisheries' closure and the government's refusal to provide compensation created anger amongst lodge owners and chaos amongst First Nations, many of whose communities descended into alcoholism and violence. In the words of Chief Andrew Rickart, "It's a sell-out of the first order, which will hurt not just my people, but all of Ontario. When Reed's greed has destroyed that forest, there will be no wilderness and eventually no timber for anyone."

Rickart stressed the long history of cooperation between his people and the settler population, but he could see that crumbling around him: "Look about you today. Are white people not ashamed? Do they not have human compassion? Do they not realize that they have literally destroyed everything we've had? All we have is our lives! Now they want that too, through greed that perpetuates cultural genocide." His eloquent plea to protect what remained of the pristine wilderness his people had inhabited for centuries, perhaps millennia, with an almost invisible footprint, fell on deaf ears, as government and industry discussed plans for another mill, this one with a start-up price of 400 million dollars and a cutting area of almost twenty thousand square miles.

Although lodge owners Marion and Barney Lamm voluntarily closed their popular fishing lodge in response to the mercury contamination, and Dr. Peter Newberry and a group of Toronto Quakers became involved, it took six years and international attention to bring non-Indigenous Ontarians onside. Dr. Harada had arranged for members of Grassy Narrows and Whitedog reserves to meet victims of Minimata disease in Japan. Jack Kent, a councillor from Whitedog, was overwhelmed by Harada's generosity and the genuine concern of his Japanese hosts: "I have been here a few days and already I have seen the governor. He is thousands of miles away. But back home, I haven't seen the government in my life. That proves their government is doing something." It also proved to him and his companions that a more radical stance needed to be taken.

According to the chief historians of this crisis, author George Hutchison and photographer Dick Wallace, whose book *Grassy Narrows* ought to be compulsory reading by all Canadians,

> At Grassy, events have tragically demonstrated how history repeats itself despite the lessons of the past. With frightening predictability, decisions have been made outside the peoples' sphere of influence and imposed upon them, creating enormous social problems which seem to intensify with the passage of time. The toll can be counted in the graveyards of Grassy.[2]

Anastasia M. Shkilnyk, who spent time in the affected communities observing and interviewing for her book, A *Poison Stronger than Love: The*

Destination of an Ojibwa Community, insists the situation could not be worse: "In this community, people have turned their anger inward, lashing out against those closest to them or against themselves. Their self-destructive response to intolerable conditions is clearly evident in the statistics on suicide."[3]

An article by Amnesty International, titled "Grassy Narrows: Provincial Inaction on Mercury Contamination Inexcusable," opens with two quotations, the first from Chief Roger Fobister Sr., of Grassy Narrows First Nation: "When we shared our land and water we expected it to be kept pristine, but they have failed and destroyed our culture as a result. We want that mercury cleaned up. There is no way around it because it is a sacred trust to take care of our land." The second quotation is attributed to Judy DaSilva, activist, health coordinator, and mother of five: "I believe some babies in our community continue to be born sick because of the mercury poison that is still in the river. These children did not choose this legacy of poisoning they have inherited." According to Amnesty International, a 2009 review commissioned by the federal and Ontario governments affirmed the fact that "high levels of mercury exposure have led to neurological disorders" amongst the people at Grassy Narrows. Moreover,

> some people continue to be exposed to high levels of mercury. The independent scientific review also noted that there was inadequate health care and support to deal with a continued health crisis affecting the community . . . The latest report, commissioned by the province and carried out by environmental scientist Patricia Sellers, found that the current contamination levels exceed the threshold established by Environment Canada for triggering an environmental cleanup in similar situations.[4]

And yet the provincial government of Kathleen Wynne refused to do anything but talk to the people and carry on with business as usual in terms of industrial development. The Grassy Narrows First Nation fears that the clear-cutting of their ancestral lands will not only leave them a wasteland and eradicate all game from the area, but also increase the mercury activity through excessive runoff. It's not difficult to understand the anger resulting from government neglect, inaction, and coziness with the corporations, not demanding higher emissions standards, not punishing the polluters for infractions, and not proceeding with cleanup.

I've turned off the radio and am listening to the sounds of wind in the tall cedars and Douglas fir around my house on Thetis Island, the clothes dryer along the hall winding down after its first rinse cycle. A comforting combo. I sit perfectly still, all ears, thinking of the deliberate refusal of public officials to listen—or, hearing, to act. A sad irony that calls up the observation from Psalm 115, verse 6: "They have ears but they hear not." The phenomenon is not new in the region. According to a 1954 report, ear experiments took place at Cecilia Jeffrey Residential School in Kenora that caused permanent hearing damage to children. Drawing from a nurse's report obtained from Indian and Northern Health Services, CBC's Jody Porter says that the smell of bad breath and discharging ears at the school was overwhelming. When not forced to irrigate their own ears with hot water, the children were subjected to a variety of experiments, including pills, nose drops, and deliberately punctured eardrums. According to nurse Kathleen Stewart, who wrote the follow-up report on the treatment of 165 students, "three were almost deaf with no ear drums, six had hearing gone in one ear."[5]

My friend and fellow poet Pam Galloway confirms in an email that this level of gross neglect was nationwide and not restricted to residential schools:

> *Your new project sounds fascinating and, yes, interests me as a health worker as well as a writer. When I first arrived in Canada many years ago, I lived in Prince George and ended up being hired to go out to Tache reserve near Fraser Lake. I was completely green, had no knowledge or understanding of First Nations. I saw some awful things like kids with ear infections so bad and untreated their ears were running with snot. I was so deeply shocked and made a complaint to various people which of course went nowhere.*

When you add this damage to the nutritional experiments conducted in six residential schools and the polio experiments performed at Goodfish Lake day-school-cum-laboratory, just for starters, it's painfully obvious that Indigenous children were considered a nuisance, but useful as guinea pigs.

Cecilia Jeffrey is the same residential school from which twelve-year-old Chanie ("Charlie") Wenjack escaped in 1966 and was found frozen to death alongside the railway tracks near Redditt, Ontario. He'd been trying to reach his home six hundred miles away. In another piece for CBC radio, a documentary called "Dying for an Education: Little Charlie," Jody Porter speaks to members of Wenjack's family, still grieving his death almost fifty years later and the failure of our society to answer the question "Why?" She also interviews journalist Ian Adams, whose article, "The Lonely Death of Charlie Wenjack," appeared in *Maclean's Magazine* in 1967. Adams had covered the coroner's inquest, where not a single Indigenous person was present or had even been notified. Adams' conclusion?

"No child should have to die like that . . . Whoever did that must have had no sense of decent humanity."[6]

Questions. But what now? Comedian Ryan McMahon understands that these events and the refusal of government to listen are not laughing matters. And Wab Kinew knows there are many reasons for walking and many paths from which to choose. But they also realize there are far too many Indigenous children, youth and adults walking wounded or, like survivors of the Rwandan genocide, moving through their days as zombies. Yes, rage destroys, but what alternative paths are provided for the wounded and the damaged, paths so desperately needed now?

thirty

Annie, Robert, and Irene

I n March 2015 I travel to Ottawa with the intention of interviewing several Elders on the subject of Indigenous health and the segregated Indian hospitals, organized around a reading I've been invited to participate in at VERSeFest, the annual Ottawa poetry festival. This is how things are done in a country the size of Canada, as the cost of air travel is prohibitive, and advances from publishers, when they are given at all, usually do not cover the costs of significant research. However, the combination serves me well in an unexpected way, as one of the participants in the same literary event is Chilean poet Raúl Zurita. I am familiar with Zurita's work and reputation from my travels to Chile during the Pinochet dictatorship.

Zurita's studies of civil engineering were interrupted by the military coup on September 11, 1973, when he was arrested, detained, tortured, and imprisoned in the hold of a naval training ship anchored in Valparaíso harbour. Much of his life and subsequent writings have been coloured by these traumatic experiences, including a period of self-mutilation and, eventually, a series of books with telling titles such as *Purgatorio* and *Anteparaiso*. These and other Dantesque works explore the descent into hell and slow return to health that were his own and Chile's experience of the dictatorship. I mention Zurita here because his is a classic case of the effects of violence and trauma on physical and mental health.

The four individuals I am meeting in the national capital area, all familiar with trauma, have been introduced to me by Métis lawyer, professor, and writer Yvonne Boyer, whom I met a year earlier. My first encounter is with Annie Smith St. Georges, an Algonquin Elder, and her husband Robert St. Georges, a Métis Elder, who live across the Ottawa River in Hull, Quebec, an urban centre now called Gatineau.

"I hope you don't mind that we both smoke," Annie says, ushering me into her small, busy kitchen. Two lovely grandsons, age seven and ten, are visiting and in the process of having a geography lesson, Robert drawing from memory a rough map of Canada and marking off the provinces and territories. Above the roar of the stove fan to eliminate the smoke, an excited budgie performs its own extended version of the welcome song.

As the intended interview had been with Annie, Robert says he will be leaving shortly. I back my car out of their driveway and park it down the street. However, we all become so engaged in the conversation that he decides to stay, offering a lively account of his life. He'd been sexually abused on a regular basis by priests in the Catholic residential school, Séminaire St-Joseph of Mont-Laurier, Quebec, that he attended as a boy. His only escape was gymnastics; in fact, he became so good he competed in several elite competitions in Canada, which could have led to a place on the Olympic team. Rage and disappointment made Robert drop out of school early and abandon his athletic dreams. His father, a singer, poet, and violin maker, had taught his son well and provided an example of hard work. Robert worked at various jobs and made violins as a hobby with his father, assisting with one that was sold to the first violinist of the Montreal symphony. She liked it so much she used it as her working instrument. This was followed by various careers, including more than a decade with the Department of Indigenous and Northern Affairs.

As we talk, Robert and Annie pass a cigarette back and forth, each taking a puff. "All that time," he says, "they never knew I was an Indian."

I do not ask Robert how he feels about that in retrospect.

On the subject of segregated Indian hospitals, Robert has little to say, but he does share a recent and very telling encounter with racism in the Canadian health-care system. After an overlong period with a bowel obstruction, he was taken to the emergency ward of a hospital in the Ottawa-Hull region, where he waited thirty-nine hours for medical attention, five hours longer than Brian Sinclair who died unattended in the emergency ward of a Winnipeg hospital.

While Robert and I exchange ideas, Annie listens quietly and engages with her grandsons as they disappear and reappear in the kitchen, doubtless hoping for the full attention of their grandparents and the rest of their interrupted geography lesson. When she finally does speak up, Annie surprises me with her passion, forthrightness, and humour. She somehow evaded residential school but not the racism that is rampant in all levels of Canadian society. Even "regular" school proved to be hell, and she paid an emotional price for her light brown skin, struggling to retain her self-confidence and ability to voice her ideas and concerns.

"My father was a strong personality," she says, "steeped in traditional knowledge. He taught me how to hunt, trap, and survive in the bush. This provided the balance I needed to survive."

So this timid child in school, who endured abuse from teachers and students alike, was nurtured at home and given many reasons to believe she was loved and worthwhile.

Annie quit school early, but her interests in dance kept her from unravelling like so many of her Indigenous contemporaries. Her skills restored her confidence and solace and brought her into contact with many talented people in the media and wider community, where she began to recover the voice silenced by the school system. One of the first things she tells me is that the Algonquin people had tried without success for two hundred years to get Ottawa to the treaty table. Now, as we speak, I can hardly believe the impressive trajectory of her life and rhetorical skills, the latter making her a special participant in the ceremonies surrounding the government's Official Apology for the residential schools. Having been asked to do the welcome, she took considerable pleasure in cordially receiving the prime minister, politicians, and guests on "unceded Algonquin territory." Afterwards, at the social gathering, the prime minister asked what she thought of his apology, to which she replied, "An apology is not an excuse, just an acknowledgement. We wait to see what your next step is."

With reluctance, I leave my chat with these strong, resilient people, planning to keep in touch and hoping to meet again.

I barely make it to the Children's Powwow at the Raven's Nest, the building that houses Carleton University's basketball team, where I am to meet Irene Lindsay. We missed our appointment the previous day because of difficult timing, as she was delayed in her work as a volunteer at the same event. I arrive at Carleton to a packed parking lot and a gymnasium of dancers in full costume—stunning beadwork, reflecting disks, feathered wings and headdresses—doing their intricate steps to the sound of drums and chanting. Irene picks me out of the crowd and whisks me off to a quiet space, where she gives me a rigorous lesson in Indigenous spiritual practices, including various uses of the Medicine Wheel and the sacred and ceremonial properties of tobacco.

Irene was born and raised in Duck Lake, Saskatchewan, where she attended Duck Lake Indian Residential School at an early age and was sexually abused repeatedly by the principal. When she turned twelve, and without asking the permission of her parents, the principal sent her to Ontario to serve as a maid and housekeeper for his friends, the motives for which one can only surmise. Irene recalls the lament of her grandmother at the station, saying, "If you go, you will lose everything." The prediction was sadly true, as language, culture, and family remained behind along with smoke from the train and the diminishing figure waving from the platform.

Her tenure did not last long with this family, a judge and his wife, apparently a former girlfriend of the principal. Irene was quickly shunted off to the household of an older couple. When the Catholic priest in Duck Lake discovered that Irene was no longer in the community, he set out to bring her back from Ontario, but ended up striking a deal with the old couple and she remained in their service. On one of her rare trips back home to attend the funeral of a sister who died of cancer at the sanatorium in Prince Albert, Irene shared stories with several female friends around a table. Apparently that same school principal had offered two of them a ride home, but instead of taking them there directly, he had shown one how to steer the car, placing a board over the accelerator and instructing her to keep the car in the middle of the long prairie road while he sexually assaulted the other sister in the back seat.

Though deeply troubled, Irene married young. I ask what impact abuse, hatred, and displacement had on her and her family.

"I had two choices," she says. "Either give in to the anger and ruin my children, or turn my back on it. I decided to raise them with love."

This was easier said than done, especially as she also coped with various illnesses until she was fifty, including gallbladder problems and chronic bleeding. After trying several diets to no avail, including multi-grains and vitamins, Irene discovered a book called *Eat Right for Your Type*, by Peter D'Adamo. The book explains that vitamin E has a tendency to make people with type-O blood bleed. His remedy was simple: return to the basic hunter-gatherer diet. Although her physical health improved, she still had not overcome the abuse and the loss of her childhood. Something was yet to happen that would to change all that.

The father of one of Irene's friends took ill and the woman spent a great deal of time caring for him in his final days. The depth of that relationship and the bonding between father and daughter had a strong impact on Irene. In spite of her decision to take the way of love with her own children, she still lacked the capacity to express grief and sadness, never having been able to cry about the loss of her own parents and sister. However, invited to attend the eventual funeral, she found herself in tears for the first time, weeping for her friend's father, heartbreaking sobs on behalf of someone she did not really know. She realized something had shifted inside her and that further healing was now necessary and possible.

That's when Irene actively set out to learn about Indigenous spiritual practice. She came to believe she was here for a purpose, that what she had learned about suffering could be put to good use. She describes attending the Star Lodge, gathering cedar twigs and boughs for the ground, observing the guides carefully sprinkling tobacco along the path, and experiencing the sweat lodge for grandmothers. It turned out to be a genuine healing experience. I'm surprised by her description of the neon effect of the tobacco sprinkled along the path as she emerged. At this point in our conversation, Irene's daughter comes to tell her mom it is time to start dismantling the crafts display. As our conversation draws to an end, Irene tells me about visiting the old residential school grounds at Duck Lake, counting twenty-one tombstones, all for children ages five to nine, and thinking to herself, "What was going on here? Schools aren't supposed to have graveyards."

221

I knew something about delayed grief, having been kept from attending the funeral of my mother as a boy of seven in Vancouver. Years later, I told a counsellor about this death and the subsequent visit of my father, who lived with a new wife in distant Saskatchewan. I was sitting at the piano, having had only twelve lessons, my father behind me on the couch smoking a cigarette. I was nervous. I desperately wanted to impress him so he would take my brother and me to live with him. As I told this story to the counsellor, I was overcome with unresolved grief, realizing in that moment that as a child I had been playing for my life and, to some degree, have been doing so ever since. If I had an Indigenous name, it would not be Dances with Wolves, but Plays for His Life.

I thank Irene and head toward the exit, where the sound of drums and singers in the gymnasium is infectious. I step inside for a few minutes to experience the final ceremonial dance, men, women, and children moving in a slow circle around the room, each doing their own unique footwork, heads of the bird-dancers bobbing, tiny costumed princesses, ecstatic, whirling amongst the throng. When the music stops, the announcer singles out a small boy for special recognition. The youngster leaves the floor with a twenty-dollar bill in his hand and a million-dollar smile lighting up his face. I join the applause and find myself weeping with joy at the spectacle.

thirty-one

Gloria in Excelsis

Gloria Nicolson, who was raised as a child on Gilford Island and the community of Gwa'yi in Kingcome Inlet, is a fluent speaker of Kwak'wala, which she has been teaching for many years, and a strong advocate of language renewal and traditional learning. According to linguist Anne Marie Goodfellow, who interviewed her and others, Gloria, like many residents of Dzawada'enuxw (Kingcome Inlet) First Nation, spent much time away, first as an involuntary guest of the Canadian government at St. Michael's Residential School in Alert Bay from age eight to the completion of grade ten. After several years living with relatives in Alert Bay, she moved at age twenty-four to Vancouver, where she completed her high school in the evenings. The period that followed included three years as a supervisor at St. Michael's, marriage, five years in Comox and many more in Vancouver, where she raised a family of five daughters and two stepchildren as well as serving as executive director of the Native Professional Women's Association. However, roots triumphed and she returned to Kingcome Inlet in the early 1990s. Back home, she worked as a teacher's aide during the regular school year and, in summer, paired elders with students who wanted to achieve greater fluency in the language.

I had the pleasure of meeting Gloria through my daughter Bronwen, who was by then community planning advisor for the Naut'sa mawt Tribal Council, a consortium of BC First Nations that included the people in Kingcome, a community 300 kilometres north of Vancouver that can best be reached by float plane, then a flat-bottomed aluminium skiff with an outboard motor that takes you the last half hour upriver east of the Broughton Archipelago, a location so beautiful and remote it gives life to the phrase "back of beyond." The nearest I'd come to Kingcome in my travels had been almost twenty years earlier, when I sailed up the coast and spent a few days at Village Island, or Mamalilikulla, the sight of the last great Potlatch, raided by the RCMP, individuals jailed, artefacts whisked away to museums and private collections. The spot where we meet, however, is anything but remote; it's the annual Elder Conference hosted this year by the Tetayut people in the Saanich Peninsula just north of Victoria, where there are so many guests I have to park a kilometre down the road. It takes Gloria and me a while to locate each other in the throng. In order to converse, we take refuge in the bleachers of the hockey arena, not far enough away to avoid the roar of voices from the craft fair in progress and a litany of corny jokes about ageing pouring from the loud-speaker next door.

Gloria tells me how fond she is of my daughter Bronwen, so I'm immediately put at ease, ready to hear about her Uncle Ernie and the bark cure, about the woman whose doctor found no TB scars in her lungs although she'd been confined to hospital for that specific disease as a child. Gloria herself spent four years as a patient in the Preventorium in Alert Bay, the medical facility attached to St. Michael's Residential School, an ugly Dickensian brick structure that I'd viewed in Alert Bay a week before it was torn down, a demolition ceremony at which former students wept uncontrollably and threw stones at the hated building to express their anger and contempt. I ask Gloria what the impact of residential school and those four sick years was like. "What I resented most about the hospital experience and the school was the years away from my parents."

The parents she regrets not spending more time with seem extraordinary as well. Her father once dismissed the theft of gasoline from his house, though he knew the identity of the thief, by rationalizing, "His family must have needed it." Her mother, too, had the gifts of patience and generosity, able to put up with gossip she did not want to hear on the grounds that the neighbour "must have needed to get it off her chest." I'm interested in knowing if she blames the school and the system for her tuberculosis. Like everyone I've spoken to so far, Gloria has had her share of negative experiences with systemic racism and prejudice from non-Indigenous institutions and people, but it's not something she chooses to dwell on. Instead, she has become fully engaged in the Kwakwaka'wakw culture and traditions, not only as a teacher of the Kwak'wala language, but also as someone involved at almost every level of life in the community, including serving as director of the local culture society. Even more significant has been her decision to make sure her children were exposed to their heritage from an early age.

According to her daughter, the celebrated visual and installation artist Marianne Nicolson, this proved to be a powerful and important experience. As she explains to interviewer Jasmine Inglis, "I had grown up on reserve and off reserve, mostly off reserve, but I would get sent home [to Gwa'yi] in the summers as a teenager, and the contrast between those cultures was so extreme, so strong, that it really marked my understanding personally." Her work as an activist or politically engaged artist, concerned not only with land claims and Indigenous rights, but also with environmental issues, is most evident in A Precarious State, a very large glass installation that has a permanent home at the Canadian Embassy in Amman, Jordan. It features a submerged killer whale with a number of characters on its back. As Marianne explains to Jasmine Inglis, "A Precarious State is pretty up front I think . . . it has this tension, you're not sure if the whale is actually being inundated by all these beings that are trying to ride on it. In my mind the whale was the land and all the beings on its back were competing interests. And then A Precarious State, you know it's a double meaning."

Judging from the Kingcome Newsletter online, there is plenty of evidence that the community is working hard to counteract isolation, racism, intergenerational trauma, and other challenges, offering news about a Health & Wellness Week, the call for a Village Clean Up, a meeting of residential school survivors to talk about available education credits, and plans to develop ecotourism. Gloria Nicolson is central to much of this activity. Unfortunately, we don't have time to talk about the oolichan runs in Kingcome Inlet or the flooding of the river that forced the people of Gwa'yi to evacuate in 2010, then put their houses on stilts, or the challenges of living so far from hospitals and the amenities. Gloria gets out when she can to visit family and friends, but is deeply committed

225

to helping improve the community. In other words, although she's at an Elder's conference, she has no intention of letting age slow her down.

Although the ambient noise and bad jokes are irritating, I am thrilled to have spent this brief time with Gloria, as her story and spirit reinforce my growing appreciation for Indigenous determination, creativity, and resilience. And the Elders Conference is another reminder of the role that humour has played in their survival. Humour releases pressure and opens doors; by turning the world upside down, it has the capacity to restore equilibrium. The subversive black humour of the Czechs helped them survive Soviet oppression, as is evidenced by the film *Closely Watched Trains* and Jaroslav Hasek's satirical novel *The Good Soldier Schweik*. So, too, Chileans survived the violence and suffering of the coup and the Pinochet dictatorship by developing various forms of black humour. As Leandro Urbina explains, one of the primary functions of the joke is to "shame people who oppose a flexible social order." He illustrates this by sharing his short-short story, "Our Father Who Art in Heaven," which highlights the theme of the innocent traitor by playing with the first line of the Lord's Prayer:

> While the sergeant was interrogating his mother and sister, the captain took the child by the hand to the other room.
> —Where is your father? he asked.
> —He's in heaven, whispered the boy.
> —What's that? Is he dead? asked the captain surprised.
> —No, said the child. Every night he comes down from heaven to eat with us.
> The captain raised his eyes and discovered the little door in the ceiling.[7]

When I interviewed Nancy, who'd had her ears, nose, and lips cut off by the Lord's Resistance Army in northern Uganda, I was outraged, wanting retribution for those who'd caused her such pain. Joseph Kony, I thought, as I retreated into my reptilian brain, a bullet is too good for you. All this while Nancy was counselling forgiveness and restoration. Nancy could see what an emotional state I was in and she graciously changed the subject. "Gary," she said, "your name is the same as the Acholi word for bicycle." I thanked Nancy and said I was glad to be mistaken for an Acholi bicycle since "Gary" in the Japanese language sounds the same as the word for diarrhea. That exchange, and the laughter it provoked, was liberating, for both of us, and for the translator.

I'm convinced that humour has been a redeeming factor for First Nations, Métis, and Inuit peoples, as evidenced by the CBC radio program *Dead Dog Café*, where Indigenous actors had a national forum from which they could make fun of the stereotypes and racist assumptions applied to them by the non-Indigenous world. Tom King wrote the script and acted in that series. He also went on to write an amazing book called *The Inconvenient Indian*, which manages to lampoon every cliché on the subject of "Indians" and their history. His book, a great success in Canada, reminded me of Tomson Highway's *The Rez Sisters*, the satirical poems by Louise (Sky Dancer) Halfe and Marilyn Dumont, and of many hilarious moments during my interviews with elders.

I'd also heard so much from those I interviewed about the importance of music, dance, and song in the recovery process that I thought I should get in touch with an Indigenous person who makes music. That's when I discovered the work of Elder Fred John in Vancouver. I tried, without success, to arrange a meeting, but managed to learn about his work through a two-part interview he'd done with David Wu in the *Caring for Our Children* newsletter.

Fred, though trained as a drug and alcohol counsellor, still felt an emptiness, something missing in his life, which drew him back to traditional cultural practices, including singing, drumming, and dancing. "I found that by singing and using the sweat lodge," he said,

> and learning more about our ways we were doing really good work for our people back home. And so I started doing the work. It came to me naturally, to learn how to sing—I must know about 100 songs in the Pow Wow way, which I try to bring in the Nations from all over, like the south, east, west and north songs when I do singing and teach the drumming.

This practice reawakened his spirit, so he thought he would share this with his people. The drum actually heals, he says, "it has the energy to clear you up and get you back in balance."[8]

In response to David Wu's question about the kind of help he offers, Fred John said:

The majority of our people don't have any idea of their own culture, so they want to learn, and they want to hear about the culture because they had a bad experience, so we help them reconnect. Once the culture is re-awakened, it's almost like the balance of their life has come back. They've been walking off-balance, like maybe you know, that something is missing. I knew I wasn't all there. I was good at what I was doing, but I didn't feel complete till I got my culture side re-awakened and brought back to me.

He also talks about the balance that can be restored by traditional practices:

There's a lot of learning to do. Sweat lodge is really a cleansing of the spirit. Not only the body—you take a shower and clean your body off, but the spirit that is in you is still not cleansed, right? It's still hurting. So what the sweat lodge does, it takes all of that, removes all of that within you.[9]

In an interview conducted by Klisala Harrison, called "Singing My Spirit of Identity: Aboriginal Music for Well-being in a Canadian Inner City," Fred John once again describes how traditional music and drumming can be meaningful, even healing, especially when he's working with poor and disadvantaged people in Vancouver's Downtown Eastside centre called The Aboriginal Front Door Society:

It makes us proud to hear the drum and the drum songs. Even though people down there would be using, they'd be drinking or doping up, when they hear the drum song, it bypasses all of that. It gets to their heart, and they will respect the drum even in that condition. They will hear it and respect it. The respect would be to walk away. They know the alcohol and drugs, they do not blend with that.[10]

The term "doctoring" that Fred John uses to describe his work with Indigenous brothers and sisters who need healing is certainly in keeping with the experience of writers, artists, and musicians in the non-Aboriginal world as well, who have found that their work has healing potential, for themselves and others. Music touches us deeply, as does her sister art, poetry. Like chant and drumming, poetry connects with those bodily rhythms, including the heartbeat, and the rhythms of eating and digesting, sleep and waking that we experience in utero and infancy. As we are weaned from the breast, language is the bridge we build back to the mother and the adult world she inhabits, a substitute umbilicus. Poetry, a primary process language, returns us to that bardo state, half asleep, half awake, during which the turmoil of the Titanic self can be processed and managed. I like what Dylan Thomas has to say about his reasons for writing poetry: "Out of the inevitable conflict of images—inevitable because of the creative, recreative, destructive, and contradictory nature of the motivating centre, the womb of war—I try to make that momentary peace which is a poem."[11]

When you've experienced the healing and wellbeing that music affords, it's not difficult to understand the terrible loss that the banning of the Potlatch and the Sundance imposed on Indigenous peoples. No wonder so many of them risked jail sentences to keep the practice alive in more remote locations. When the RCMP raided the last great Potlatch on the west coast at Mamalilikulla, or Village Island, in 1935, the practice did not end, but shifted deeper inland amongst forests, inlets, and river systems such as those at Gwa'yi, Gloria Nicolson's home-place.

Laughter, the arts, and music, which have helped to heal Indigenous people through the trials by fire of displacement, residential schools, and segregated hospitals, are definitely important medicines for the road ahead. I know they've sustained me along this very difficult and challenging path, even when I can' t understand the imagery or lyrics and when the humour is at my own expense. I don't mind admitting, at the risk of being dismissed as a sentimental slob, that this journey through the minefields of Indigenous health care is putting me more in touch not only with Canada's disturbing political realities, but also with my own emotions, including anger and grief at the unresolved loss I spoke of in the previous chapter. It's an unexpected gift for which I am increasingly grateful.

As Gloria and I vacate our not-exactly-quiet corner, the parting joke blasting from the speakers is attributed to Woody Allen: "It's not that I'm afraid to die. I just don't want to be there when it happens."

229

thirty-two

Albert, Racism, and Anger

Yvonne Boyer, whom I mentioned earlier, a lawyer from the Saskatchewan Métis Nation with a practice in Ottawa, has a background that includes nursing and serving on the Aboriginal Healing Foundation. I met her briefly in Ottawa and had the pleasure of reviewing her book, *Moving Aboriginal Health Forward: Discarding Canada's Legal Barriers* in the *Vancouver Sun*. Her research interested me because it covered much of the same ground as my own, but from a legal and constitutional angle, the premise being that if Indigenous people are considered second-class citizens and kept at a distance and disadvantage, their health will continue to suffer.

"The failure of Aboriginal health policies," as she says in the introduction, "resides in the false assumptions that Aboriginal people were biologically predetermined to vanish, were inherently unhealthy and inferior, and that their culture causes them to pursue harmful lifestyles."[12]

In outlining the determinants responsible for the bad health of Aboriginal peoples in Canada, she focuses on stress and poverty:

The body breaks down as stresses compound and intensify. Under these conditions, the options for sustaining healthy lifestyles and the ability to acquire help in health crises narrow. Illness and death are far more likely for those who are poor and marginalized. People who are not marginalized, who are not living in poverty, who enjoy adequate housing, who are educated, and whose cultural identity is not under attack have better states of health.[13]

The statistics that back up this situation are alarming. In 1924, Indigenous peoples were 1/22nd of the population, but accounted for one-quarter of the deaths. As Boyer puts it,

> health policies were geared toward protecting the good health of non-Aboriginal people. Aboriginal women have always faced social, economic, political and cultural changes that negatively affected health, cultural identity, and social and family structures. Years of assimilation have led to the medicalization of birthing and the decline of traditional midwifery practice.[14]

Although Boyer is concerned with exposing the legal impediments to good Indigenous health, it's clear that systemic racism has shaped and maintained the legislation that bedevils positive change. When Allan and Smylie's report, *First Peoples, Second Class Treatment: The Role of Racism in the Health and Well-being of Indigenous Peoples in Canada*, was released in 2015, Boyer was one of the first academics to respond. After emphasizing that Indigenous people's rights to adequate health care are guaranteed not only in the Charter of Rights, but also in the treaties, she offers a spirited and impassioned argument in support of the report's conclusions about racism that confirms much of what I'd been learning during the previous four years:

> These documents affirm the right to health and health care as an important part of Canada's agreement with the First Peoples. But yet, we hear of Indigenous people in Canada dying in emergency rooms and being ignored by some health care professionals who assume the Aboriginal clients seeking help are homeless and looking for a "free ride" in their emergency room. Such incidences, rather than reinforcing the role of care that grounds the health care system and its providers, perpetuate the injustices suffered by the most vulnerable of the vulnerable—the homeless and others who are sexually exploited or involved in sex work on the streets.

Research has shown time and again that historical and complex socioeconomic issues for many Indigenous people in Canada have resulted from racism, including the legacy of physical and sexual abuse experienced in the residential school system, dispossession of identity and culture via the Indian Act, violence, and the marginalization of Indigenous women. These racial attacks on cultures and nations of Peoples undermine cultural knowledge, attack self-esteem, promote poverty, and create a heightened vulnerability to being trafficked as human beings. Experts, who have lived the experiences and were canvassed for the 2014 Public Safety Canada Report, "Trafficking of Aboriginal Women and Girls," were clear that racist experiences were a strong element, if not the overarching theme, in the experiences of vulnerable women when accessing health care. Stories told and retold were experiences of racism, including routinely asked questions such as, "How much have you had to drink?" "What drugs have you done?" and "You are a prostitute, are you not?" These vulnerable women told of the horrors of being trafficked and raped and having to endure the smack of racism from cold responses, racial questioning and refusal of care. Some of the women learned to rely upon a trusted advocate to ensure the violence they endured would be taken seriously by the health care system. There was a perception that the nursing staff hoped the woman would just go away. Indeed, women do often get tired of waiting, go back to a shelter and do not return to the hospital and the rape goes unreported.[15]

It was with these thoughts in mind that I set out to interview the last of the Quebec and Ontario contacts Boyer had given me. Albert Dumont, who had made it only to grade seven, left school and Catholicism behind at age twelve to pursue his career as a bricklayer. He had managed to avoid residential school, but not the heavy hand of racist attitudes and practices from staff and students at his public school. Alcohol was his constant companion during the following years, a thin, unreliable mortar barely holding together the shaky building blocks of a troubled self. Because he was such a good bricklayer, however, his occasional absences were tolerated, and eventually he hired his own crew. As he walked me through those troubled years, he paused to show me photographs of his beautiful daughters. Albert finally gave in to the need for counselling and healing and tells me, proudly, that he has been sober for twenty-seven years.

When I bring up the subject of racism, Albert gets quite heated about the disparaging views of First Nations expressed by Sun TV's adversarial broadcaster, Ezra Levant.

"I don't understand why he makes these comments about us. The Jews elected their first politician as early as 1807 in Lower Canada, then another in 1836 in Upper Canada. Meanwhile, we were denied the vote until 1960. If we'd had the vote a hundred years earlier there would have been no residential schools."

I love the slight Irish lilt and accent in Albert's speech, the th-sounds often emerging as a single t-sound.

"Things have got to change," he says. "It's greed. People, in their subconscious, if another group with a lower status rises up, understand it will mean a change in their standard of living. That's why there's so much resistance to Obama and what he represents. There'll be a lot of bloodshed down there, as the black people won't stand for repression much longer. Something's gotta give."

I marvel aloud that Indigenous anger has so consistently turned inward on the self, the family, and the community rather than outward to the settler population.

"I've got this friend," Albert says, standing up to check the moose-meat pie in the oven, "who can say what he wants to me. Same as I can say what I want to him. He's talking about a Native protest and road-block and says: 'I'd just take the biggest, meanest gun I could find and blow them all right off the road!' So I says to him, 'Suppose you are away from your house for more than a month and when you come back there is this family living in your house. So, you say, *What the hell are you doing in my house?* And they say, *Well, in our land if someone vacates their house for more than thirty days anyone can take it.* So you get your friends with signs outside the house and begin to protest this occupation. And that guy gets a hold of the biggest, meanest gun he can find and blows the lot of you right off the road."

"What was his response?

"He never said a word."

I describe for Albert being at a protest the previous week in Victoria against the Conservative government's Anti-Terrorism Act, Bill C-51, where a good portion of the crowd of a thousand or more are Indigenous people. An Elder from the Cowichan Nation comes up to the mike and says, "This bill is about terrorism. Well, we've been fighting terrorism here since the 1400s." The crowd goes crazy with applause.

Albert laughs. "That's my father there," he says, pointing to a striking photograph taped to the fridge door, the face strong, clear-eyed, and confident. "He was a highly respected lumberjack. He married my mother, had some kids. When we moved from Kitigan Zibi, an Anishinaabeg reserve in Quebec, he was working for John Sherwin, the original owner of Sherwin-Williams Paints. Four major families in the new town signed a document saying it was okay for us to live in this white community, but other folks were not so sympathetic. They came at night, tossed rocks through the windows and shouted: 'Go back where you came from, you goddam Indians.' Imagine that, we were right in the heart of our own community and they told us to go back where we came from. We had a good work ethic, we were respected, and we were devout Christians. So I ask the question, whenever I'm invited to give a talk, why would they want to drive us out? It's racism, pure and simple. I tell people this, and it's as if they're hearing it for the first time. We had no freedom. We had to get a white man to sign a paper saying we could spend time outside the reserve. They didn't want any one interfering with their rape and pillage of the land. The early settlers were driven by greed, the desire to get something for nothing."

Remembering Robert St. George's comment about the AFN, I ask Albert if he thinks this organization of chiefs has failed its mandate.

"There's some very able leaders. Where else do you find a guy like Ovide Mercredi? He came to our protests and marched with us. Even in the old days when there were only about a dozen or so, there he was alongside us. As we get more and more educated and confident, things will have to change. The early chiefs competed for advantage, so the government just ignored us. Chief Partridge, a great leader amongst the Algonquin, petitioned the government for decades to sign a treaty, but was just ignored.

The Parliament buildings are on stolen land. Do people understand that? We brought the bible here, they say, as if that's the big consolation prize. It's enough to make your head swim."

Much of our subsequent conversation circles around issues of Indigenous spirituality and healing, including blanket ceremonies, where the troubled individual is wrapped in public in a special blanket and embraced by friends, all of whom pray for his or her healing, committing themselves to helping with the process. Albert's own healing journey has led to positive work in the community, including Millhaven Penitentiary, where he instituted a Harmony Circle to work with 130 hardened criminals to reduce violence. This involved bringing together the head honchos of the Christian, Muslim, Indian, Asian, Hell's Angels, and other gangs, not an easy challenge and one that had scared off many willing counsellors already. These men were among the most violent offenders in a community that employed brutal physical force, even putting arsenic in food that caused three days of excruciating pain before achieving its desired effect. The convicts, however hardened, were often afraid to eat. Somehow, Albert was able to command both attention and respect, significantly reducing the number and intensity of violent acts in prison.

At the moment, he's a regular at 510 Rideau Street in Ottawa, a centre for the homeless, many of whom are members of Ottawa's three thousand–strong Inuit community. The city and the former Conservative government withdrew support from this organization, another sign that their Official Apology was as hollow as a dried-out gourd. As Albert serves up large portions of moose pie, I mention the names of half a dozen Indigenous writers I respect and the prizes they were winning, including poet Louise (Sky Dancer) Halfe, who was just named poet laureate of Saskatchewan.

"I've got a friend named Phil Jenkins, a journalist," Albert tells me. "He's English, but has been around this area for thirty years. Phil's a supporter of Aboriginal rights. He sees the change coming, just like the Irish did when they started to produce the world's greatest English-speaking writers."

There are a lot of laughs as we exchange anecdotes and talk about restorative justice issues, the corrections system, and his cottage on the shore of a remote lake. My favourite among Albert's stories concerns Little George, a bricklayer he hired who had a drinking problem.

"I could handle that," Albert said, "since I had one too. But I told him he'd have to work alone on jobs, mix his own mortar. One day a big Indian guy named Darren from up north joined the crew. Little George borrowed ten dollars from him and promised to pay it back, but at the end of the week he collected his pay and skipped town. Darren says to me: 'If you see that little bugger, tell him if I ever catch him I'm going to make hamburger out of him.' Well, sure enough, I encounter him in a bar one day and pass on the message, to which Little George replies: 'Oh yeah, just ten dollars worth of hamburger?'"

As I say goodbye to Albert, I think again of Raúl Zurita, of the trauma he and Chile experienced under the coup and dictatorship. What happened to the Indigenous peoples of Canada, no less traumatic, was not a coup, but a cancer, slow-moving at one time, galloping at another. Even now, the cancer has not been cured. As I fly home, I begin reading the two books of his poetry and stories that Albert gave me as a parting gift, *Of the Trees and Their Wisdom* and *Broad Winged Hawk*. Amongst the celebrations of the natural world, there are engaged poems about racism and the activism needed to confront it. Albert asks us to imagine how a child in residential school, torturer on one side, paedophile on the other, could maintain the will to survive. And in a disturbing revision of the national anthem, which addresses the terrible death toll of residential school children, he poses two essential questions:

O Canada
Over fifty thousand children died
Their deaths are a tumour
On your soul as a nation
What doctoring will remove it
Are you not ashamed[16]

236

thirty-three

Northern Ontario Visions ─────────────────────────

"It's not easy being green," says Kermit the Frog on *Sesame Street*. If you
ask an Indigenous person in Canada, it's even less easy, and not very
good for your mental health, being invisible. These thoughts come to me
as I spend my first few days in Sault Ste. Marie in the wilds of northwestern
Ontario, where the government has found Indigenous people so easy to
ignore.

The myth of the empty land has been difficult to eradicate, and some
of our best poets have subscribed to that myth, out of ignorance or indifference. In 1948, Douglas LePan announced that he lived in "A Country
Without a Mythology," though there were Indigenous people around,
whom he referred to as "savage people, masks / Taciturn or babbling out
an alien jargon," but apparently not inviting enough to merit contact or
serious attention. The land was scarily empty with "struggling roots," "hys-
terical birds," and "weeds that clutch at the canoe." "Who will stop," he
asks rhetorically, "where, clumsily contrived, daubed / With war-paint,
teeters some lust-red manitou."[17] I'm not sure why the Algonquin or his forest and life force have such erotic connotations for the poet, and why the
former is teetering, unless the suggestion is that he's been into the sauce
newly introduced by Europeans.

Earle Birney's poem "Canlit" addresses what he considered to be
Canada's short, empty history, penning the line, "It's only by our lack of
ghosts we're haunted."[18] Was he near-sighted or constantly getting lost in the

bush? At least Frank Scott, dean of law at McGill University and one of the drafters of the Regina Manifesto that launched and defined the CCF, the socialist league that eventually morphed into the New Democrats, must have known better. However, we find him, in a poem called "Laurentian Shield," announcing a "huge silence," a land "Inarticulate, arctic, / Not written on by history, empty as paper." This land, the speaker says, "will choose its language / When it has chosen its technic," which suggests a culture based on industrial activity and not exactly "A language of flesh and roses."

Frank Scott's poem, subtly crafted, shifts emphasis halfway through, when the clever word-play of "Cabin syllables, / Nouns of settlement / Slowly forming with steel syntax" brings us to "The long sentence of its exploitation." A lawyer does not use the words "sentence" and "exploitation" without a keen awareness of their various connotations. Thus, "a deeper note" sounds in the poem, though still without reference to any Indigenous presence, acknowledging the inevitable "culture of its occupation." You could call this poem a paean to our industrial future, were it not for those three words of caution: "sentence," "exploitation," and "occupation." The final line, which prophesies millions turning rock into children, strikes a menacing note for me, when I think of the damage done to this land and the thousands of Indigenous children and adults turned into dust by a racist, colonial, industrial vision.[19]

No mythology, no ghosts, the land silent and empty? I spend one Saturday travelling west from Sault Ste. Marie to Agawa with Tom O'Flanagan, a visual artist teaching at Algoma University, to see the pictographs on a cliff face along the north shore of Lake Superior. It is a stunning landscape, where the great lake overwhelms, or at least challenges, the great shield of Precambrian rock that extends mostly unimpeded from the northern prairies into the eastern Arctic to include portions of Quebec and Greenland. Talk about geologic history; this is ancient land, part of a continent 2.5 billion years old, its thin layer of soil not much good for agriculture, but rich in minerals and capable of supporting large numbers of wild animals, including moose, deer, bear, wolves, mink, weasels, wolverines, turtles, and that shy, buck-toothed national symbol, the beaver, who, despite its good ecological reputation, shares our propensity for damming rivers and streams and cutting down trees.

The ancient rock paintings, thirty-five in number on ten panels, mostly ochre-red in colour, have faded over the centuries, but are a stunning record of earlier times, visions, and dreams, some possibly three hundred years old, including abstract shapes, a horse, a canoe with several paddlers, an eagle, a bear, a turtle, and one spectacular mythical, horned, dinosaur-like aquatic monster known as Mishipeshu, capable of calming or stirring the waters. Although these pictographs were not seen by a non-Indigenous person until 1958, their presence was already known, having been described and drawn for an Indian Agent, who would never get to see them, by Anishinaabe Chief Shingwaukonse about a century earlier, the same chief who would request a "big teaching wigwam" for his people. It is this wigwam that brings me to Sault Ste. Marie.

This evening Tom and his wife meet me at the former factory building downtown that has been renovated and turned into an arts centre, also housing Algoma University's Department of Fine Art. A new documentary film about the Group of Seven called *Painted Land* is being screened, recounting the search by Gary and Joanie McGuffin and art historian Michael Burtch to locate the original sites of famous paintings by Tom Thomson, Lawren Harris, A.Y. Jackson, Frederick Varley, Arthur Lismer, and the others. The transformed factory was packed, the circular upper balcony lined with blow-ups of the First World War paintings by these men when they were war artists that still pack a devastating punch, especially Varley's wagonload of war dead entitled *For What?* and A.Y. Jackson's ironically titled *A Copse: Evening*, which portrays the bombed-out wreckage of no-man's land with its mounds of earth, water-filled craters, and a few soldiers passing through in the distance, mud-spattered, little more than irrelevant vertical extensions of the blasted earth. Perhaps it was the ugliness and senselessness of human slaughter that drove these men into the pristine wilderness, where the human presence was not absent, but at least minimal. The film honours that vision, using several still photographs of the original group at work in the wild and some moving bits of text from their correspondence.

I am touched by the film and its intent and by the beauty and lure of the landscape. But I am reminded again of the difference between photography and painting, the latter a medium that has always seemed to me more subjective, involving more interpretation and manipulation, the blank canvas and the developing use of space, light, and colour demanding something other than what the eye has seen and more of what it is now confronting during the process of creation and recall. However, I am surprised to see no mention of the Indigenous presence either in the Group of Seven paintings or in the film itself, not even a passing reference to the pictographs of Agawa. Did the Group of Seven painters see the land as empty? Fortunately, after the screening someone in the audience poses the question forming in my mind: "Is there any sense of an Aboriginal presence in their work?" The chief spokesperson for the film fumbles with this one, saying of course the Group must have been aware of Indigenous people, making use of their skills as guides. It is an unintentionally telling remark about our ongoing relations with First Nations, Inuit, and Métis that they are invisible except when useful.

Later, looking back on this day, I come across a link to the 2007 NFB documentary *The Invisible Nation*, directed by Richard Desjardin and Robert Monderie, which recounts the historical dislocation of the Algonquin peoples and the theft and plundering of their land, driven from the Ottawa Valley north and east, and depicts current conditions in ten remote communities, most of them desolate, impoverished, dysfunctional, living in miniscule reserves, betrayed by both the federal government and the government of Quebec, the latter having refused to sign any treaties acknowledging Aboriginal title. It's a powerful and shocking reminder of what we have done to the original inhabitants of this land, viewing them as beneath contempt and rendering them virtually invisible.

My motive for being in northern Ontario is quite the opposite. I'm here not to explore a supposedly empty land, though I, too, can appreciate its beauty. My purpose is to meet and interview some of the flesh-and-blood individuals who have been so notably missing in art and literature, at least until recently when a host of Indigenous activists and writers burst into view and prominence. While doing a few literary gigs for Algoma University and waiting for word-of-mouth contacts with Elders to materialize, I spend the spare minutes during my visit to The Soo devouring a copy of Joseph Boyden's *Three Day Road*, given to me by Judith Mountjoy, the landlady of Creekside Terrace B&B in Regina, when I complained that

I couldn't find a copy in town. I'm reading a sizeable chunk of the book on the beach at Batchawana Bay, halfway between The Soo and Agawa, engrossed in the story while my faculty host, Rob Rutherdale, pours over his course notes and marking.

Sunlight reflects off the light chop and the rhythm of waves breaking on the shore of Lake Superior provides an antidote to the scenes on the page, where the World War I Cree veteran Xavier inhabits two worlds: the disorientation of PTSD, brought on by deafness, years of killing, loss of a leg, and the death of his bosom pal Elijah; and recurring nightmares of the killing fields, where he has functioned as a deadly sniper at the Somme and Vimy Ridge, using his skills as a northern Ontario hunter to outsmart and exterminate the enemy. The irony here, more apparent to a contemporary reader than to Xavier, is that his real enemy is back home, where people like him live without even human status as "persons" in what amounts to an ethnic concentration camp, deprived of rights, land, and dignity. Instead, he focuses on the Canadian bombardment being unleashed on the German trenches and the screaming shells, the body fragments flying through the air. Later, when the Canadians are being mowed down, he thinks of his aunt Kiska back home, whispering her name over and over. Then the link, as if I had not noticed where I am: "I realize as I stumble and fall to my knees that the sound of waves crashing is my own breathing."[20]

At this moment on the beach at Batchawana Bay, nature and art are in cahoots, at least in terms of wave action. And the realization also comes to me that being a professional sniper in a foreign hell-hole was not only an escape from being an Indigenous person in Canada, but also the sole means open to Xavier at the time of proving his worth as a person and becoming, however briefly, visible.

thirty-four

Mike, Ed, Alice, and the Tenuous Connection_____

From the earliest days of this research, it's been my view that the residential schools and segregated Indian hospitals were intimately linked. I stated in the brochure I printed and handed out at the TRC hearings in 2013 that residential schools served as farm teams or recruiting grounds for the Indian hospitals, ensuring that available beds remained full and providing fresh fodder for medical research. Many of the students who ended up in the segregated hospitals had been infected in the schools, either deliberately or as a result of neglect, forced to sit in the classroom alongside someone with open sores or thrown in the sickroom as punishment and obliged to share a bed with an infected child. If you weren't compliant, or you openly objected to being separated from your parents, beaten, or used as a sexual object, watch out. Those years spent in the hospitals should have been part of the compensation process. So it was with great excitement that I read CBC journalist Jody Porter's reports about just such a case, in northern Ontario, being mounted against the federal government.

Mike Cachagee, involved in this effort for redress on behalf of survivors of the Fort William Sanatorium, has agreed to meet me for lunch. Active in the Chapleau Cree First Nation, Mike is engaged in the fields of education, governance, land claims, and health as well as serving as chief of his community at Fox Lake and political advisor to the Grand Chief of the Nishnawbe Aski Nation. When we meet at a truck stop restaurant on the Trunk Road through Sault Ste. Marie, Mike is quick to insist that a balance has to be struck between abuse that happened at the residential school and the safe and secure feelings survivors have about their association with the Bishop Fauquier Memorial Chapel. I'm not sure exactly what he means, having just wandered through the lightly forested area around the university and come upon the "official" Shingwauk cemetery, which is definitely not big enough to account for the 100 to 150 deaths of students who attended that school. The cemetery does not even contain a list of names of those who died there, although many of them are said to be recorded in the Memorial Chapel.

One of Mike's most touching stories was told to him by a man who watched from a safe distance as his brother and other children were loaded into a plane and flown away to attend residential school, the plane aloft and becoming smaller and smaller until it was no more than a dot in the sky, then vanishing. Although the plane delivered its cargo of kids safely, the man's brother never returned. There was more than a single message embedded in this anecdote, one of which is that the white man's technology is much more advanced than his sense of morality and justice.

Only four and a half when he was sent to residential school, Mike spent the next twelve years there, with never a holiday or a hug. Back home, his mother had remarried and started another family and was estranged from her teenaged son. A few weeks after we meet for lunch, Mike will be interviewed in his fight against enforcing the deadline for children of residential school survivors to apply for the special education credits that were part of the government's Independent Assessment Process. Mike wants to share these credits among three grand children in post-secondary education, but this is not allowed. Before we part, he promises to introduce me to key members of the community, including former Shingwauk students and his co-worker on the redress file.

One of the prime movers Mike mentioned in the preparation of the redress is Ed Sadowski, who has picked me up in Sault Ste. Marie and is taking me east to his place on the St. Mary River. As the sign on an abandoned railway trestle—THIS IS INDIAN LAND—suggests, it's not only one of the more picturesque regions of the Canadian Shield, bordering the Great Lakes, but also contested land. After picking me up in town, Ed insists on stopping to show me the site of the original Shingwauk school at Garden River, a few kilometres east of Sault Ste. Marie, a building that subsequently burned to the ground, perhaps a result of arson, and offering his speculations about who might be buried on the site.

As we glide between the islets and rocky outcrops in his small runabout, Ed explains to me that the RFD, Request for Direction, for the segregated hospital case has been filed. He's hopeful but cautious, knowing how long such decisions can take and also the efforts that will be made by government and church lawyers to defeat such a case should it receive funding and approval to proceed. Ed's no slouch. He is an activist who completed a graduate degree in Development Studies at London School of Economics and who has worked in many fields, on assignment as a communications engineer/consultant to the Moazmbique News Agency and as a United Nations Electoral Official representing Canada to supervise Mozambique's first (free and fair) presidential and parliamentary elections in 1994. Until recently, he was an adjunct professor in the Department of Politics and Law at Algoma University. He has had a long association with the Children of Shingwauk Alumni Association, coordinating their archives and visiting centre at the university and working with the National Residential School Survivors Society.

In addition to giving me his unique perspective on Algoma University and its struggle to create a positive meeting ground for the Indigenous and non-Indigenous communities in northern Ontario, so much at the whim and wisdom of constantly changing administrators, he is also well steeped in the history of the area. We're sharing this excursion with Ed's dog, Buddy, nose pressed forward in the bow, clearly bored with our discussion and on the lookout for more interesting signs of life as we pass through what seems to be a navigational obstacle course, the ragged shoreline dotted with every kind of waterfront dwelling, from modest cottages and log houses to pretentious structures at odds with the setting, each with its long private dock stretching out through the reeds towards deeper water.

The premise for the case being mounted in Ontario is slightly different from what I'd expected. Ed and his clients claim that because the Indigenous students at the Fort William Sanatorium were being taught while in hospital, their experience was essentially the same as that of residential school students, the similarity even more obvious when you realize, in Ed's words, that because of "the shortages of beds at sanatoriums and hospital schools, residential schools received a subsidy of 15 cents per day per student for each student who had TB. Some residential schools had TB case rates as high as 80 per cent, becoming de facto sanatoriums." Along with the previous quotation in CBC journalist Jody Porter's piece, "Indian hospital survivors want Hospital added to the residential school settlement agreement," are some telling words from medical historian Maureen Lux, who points out that not only did Indian Affairs pay for the teachers and books in the hospitals and sanatoria, but also "there was a kind of seamlessness between institutions." All this, of course, happened while there was an official prohibition from Indian Affairs against allowing, or keeping, infected students in the residential schools.

Should the RFD be approved, government lawyers will try to deny that similarity, insisting that education in the hospitals amounted to nothing more than day-school training, already declared ineligible. However, Mike Cachagee counters that argument by insisting that, as sick kids and wards of the state, the patients were essentially captives. They could not say no or go home at night. It's worth noting, too, in this connection, that a case has been mounted to include day schools in the compensation process, since so many of them were staffed by racists and abusers.

Pine Island, where Ed and his wife Kelly live, is part of a group of islands, including the larger St. Joseph Island, that were common stopping places during the fur trade, a respite from the immensity and exposure of two great lakes, as well as being contested ground during the US–Canada boundary disputes. Both islands found themselves on the Canadian side, but so close to the international boundary that simple excursions like ours could mean frequent sovereignty violations. The final border resolution struck me as symbolic of the situation that now prevails between Indigenous and non-Indigenous peoples, where boundaries are constantly being called into question, especially when it comes to rights, freedoms, and land claims.

As Ed deftly manoeuvres his craft back to its berth at the dock, I try to keep Buddy from leaping out too soon and ending up in the drink, a possible destination for me as well. Alice Ridout, who lives on nearby

St. Joseph Island with her husband, has offered to take me back to town, where she has a meeting or evening class to teach at Algoma, a gesture that will save Ed a second trip to The Soo. While we wait for her, Ed serves tea and biscuits and explains how his place morphed from a humble cabin into such a gorgeous dwelling, with the spatial exorbitance of a small cathedral. To my surprise, he also informs me that a similar case involving the Indian hospitals is being prepared in western Canada and that Roy Little Chief of the Siksika Reserve in southern Alberta is one of the spokespersons. I'd talked with Roy on the phone months earlier and he had not mentioned the plan, a humbling reminder of how tenuous my connections still are within the Indigenous community.

On the way back to The Soo, Alice, who grew up in England, tells me that when she and her husband first came to Canada, they lived on the mainland across from Pine Island and used to take their dog for runs there. She laughs when I mention the narrow one-lane man-made causeway to the island, and remembers how amused they were by the signs at both ends that read: Give Way to Oncoming Traffic.

"It gave us images of super-polite Canadians waiting all day for each other to cross!"

Alice has been the dynamo behind my brief residency at Algoma University, tirelessly working out a schedule and lodging and guiding me through the ethics review process required for anyone associated with the university who is doing research with Indigenous peoples. A few months later, she writes to me of a painful Christmas visit to the UK, where her mother's Alzheimer's symptoms were devastating: "Not only do you have to cope with the loss of that person but seeing a human subject just unravel like that is so disturbing. You see just how much story holds us together as people in the world and when you cannot remember your own story you are lost."

It's a profound and moving comment that goes right to the core of what she does so effectively as a human being and as a teacher of literature and what I and so many others are trying to do, struggling against cultural amnesia, gathering and honouring the Indigenous stories that give us all a deeper meaning as Canadians and bring us closer together.

thirty-five

Shirley and the Shingwauk Project

When I attended the hearings of the TRC in Victoria's Empress Hotel in April, 2012, I did not pay much attention to the helpers situated strategically in readiness around the auditorium with their boxes of facial tissues and words of solace. However, as I listen to the shared experiences of survivors of residential schools and Indian hospitals and of so many stories everyday racism across the country, I am constantly reminded of how deep some of these wounds are. Milan Kundera was describing all of us, Indigenous and non-Indigenous alike, when he wrote, "It takes so little so infinitely little, for a person to cross the border beyond which everything loses meaning: love, conviction faith, history. Human life—and herein lies the secret—takes place in the immediate proximity of that border, even in direct contact with it; it is not miles away, but a fraction of an inch."[21]

I learned early on that word-of-mouth contact would be the only way of establishing the kind of trust that makes the sharing of experiences possible. A hundred emails or phone calls to tribal offices did not result in a single interview, but the recommendation of someone who trusted me and considered me reliable had the potential to open doors. So this has been my way of proceeding, at times frustratingly slow. Knowing that Indigenous peoples have been waiting a long time for us to listen to them, I pressed on, asking each new contact for help. Moving slowly has allowed me to mature in terms of understanding the conditions affecting Indigenous people and how these conditions have not only shaped and damaged their lives, families, and communities, but also, in

247

some notable instances, resulted in them developing incredible strengths and achievements. There is much to be said about the benefits of chance and serendipity in this kind of research, discouraging the kind of inductive reasoning that seeks only evidence to prove a pre-existing theory and keeping me open to illumination and surprise.

This was how I came to meet Shirley Horn in Sault Ste. Marie. The previous fall my wife Ann Eriksson and I had done a cross-Canada joint book promotion tour that included a visit to Algoma University. After we read in the auditorium, someone asked me about my latest project. When I explained that I was gathering information about segregated Indian hospitals, as well as their links to residential schools, the incoming dean Richard McCutcheon asked if I realized I'd just read my work in the auditorium of the former Shingwauk Residential School, which had been incorporated into the building plan of Algoma University. This was a shock. I had a copy of J.R. Miller's *Shingwauk's Vision: A History of Native Residential Schools* on my shelf at home, but thus far had only skimmed it. Then the dean-to-be suggested we try to arrange another visit, during which I could access their Shingwauk archives and First Nations contacts in exchange for a reading, a lecture, and possibly a creative writing seminar.

In September 2015, I headed east, stopping first in Regina to talk to Lorraine Yuzicapi as well as Bill Asikinack, two of whose sisters had been students at Shingwauk Residential School. By the time I arrived in The Soo, I knew that a school had been requested as early as 1832 by Chief Shingwaukonse, a "big teaching wigwam" for his people, and that request, renewed by his son, was eventually granted in 1871. Along with the school came a young English cleric named E.F. Wilson, who would serve as Shingwauk's first principal. J.R. Miller provides a stunning account of the Shingwauk Reunion in 1991, 120 years after the establishment of the school, during which former students shared their traumas, disappointments, joys, and complicated memories in the presence of politicians, bureaucrats, and a former missionary, whose attempt to justify the abusive, underfunded, and racist institution was condescending in the extreme. Here is Miller's description of that event:

> The feature of the Shingwauk reunion that promised the most constructive outcome, both for the gathering itself and for

the entire residential school experience, was the point that the chief of Garden River made on the first afternoon. Chief Darrel Boisonneau argued that residential schools were an experiment in cultural genocide that should never have taken place, and he contended that Indians needed a healing process to get over the damage that was done to them by these schools. Part of that process involved taking control of their own lives and well-being. And part of that self-empowerment, in turn, was the assumption of control of Native education by Native peoples. The land on which the reunion was talking place, he reminded his audience, was Indian land: not government or church property, but Ojibwa land. And he promised that on this land there would arise an Indian post-secondary institution that would reflect aboriginal values and be controlled by Indians. Such a university would be, he said, 'the true realization of Chief Shingwauk's vision of a 'teaching wigwam.' In 1981 and 1991, former students had come to Algoma College as guests. At the next reunion in 2001, Chief Boissoneau declared, they would come to their own institution— to Shingwauk University.[22]

While the prophecy has not been fulfilled exactly as anticipated, Shingwauk University exists within the present structure of Algoma University, much as Victoria College and St. Michael's College exist within the larger structure of the University of Toronto.

Mike Cachagee has come through as promised, arranging for me to meet Shirley Horn during the last of my twelve days at Algoma University. He tells me nothing about Shirley in advance, so I go into the interview ignorant, except for the assumption that she's a Shingwauk survivor. I wonder how she feels about being in this institution and in my temporary office in the bowels of the library, with its single window and unusual décor, including the copy of an ancient map of Iceland, in which the cartographer's depiction of surfacing whales, based only on hearsay, shows some of them with two blow-holes and what look more like long tresses than steam blowing out.

Shirley shows no signs of discomfort. In fact, she seems more at home here than I am.

"I live with my sister who is eighty on the Missanabie Cree First Nation, a tiny community of just thirty people, with all the usual hardships of winter, especially when you burn wood," she explains.

I point to the cookies and coffee on the desk.

"Is it black?" When I shake my head, she beams. "Wonderful, that's how I like it, with cream."

"A lucky guess," I say, "except it's milk instead of cream." After some small talk, it turns out we have at least one other location in common—Yorkton, Saskatchewan, where I spent a few years as a kid on a nearby farm, hoeing potatoes and gathering Seneca root along the road allowances in summer, which I later sold for a pittance to a herbalist in town.

"I worked in the hospital in Yorkton in geriatrics," Shirley says. "My husband ran a bakery there in '71 and '72."

I learn that she was raised in Chapleau, Ontario, and went to St. John's Residential School before transferring at age seven to Shingwauk, where she spent six years. She tells me she has no experience with the segregated hospital system, so our talk shifts to the subjects of racism and restorative justice. I tell Shirley a bit about my research in Africa, including Nancy's amazing capacity to forgive the abducted boys who mutilated her and to recommend restoring them to the community.

"That's my belief, too," Shirley says. "That's how I feel about the residential schools. I'm on the other side of the experience now. I'm looking through a different lens. If we're truly going to believe the teachings—the grandfather teachings in our case, or the scriptural teachers in the Christian religion, the spirit of Jesus without all the trappings—*that's* what we need to do. And it's not easy."

I tell her about Joanie Morris and her mom's long stay in the Nanaimo Indian Hospital and am surprised by her answer.

"They had a goal, which was to wipe out the Native population. And they did it blatantly, with the blankets at first, smallpox blankets introduced into the communities. Why wouldn't they, especially if it was government policy."

I tell her of my initial doubt about smallpox blankets, then finding Tom Swanky's book on the subject, and learning about the two years of missing records in Governor Douglas's office.

"Why would those records be missing?" Shirley's question is rhetorical, but it seems to require a response.

"Swanky's a lawyer. He had the determination and the patience to track it all down."

There's a pause, then Shirley says, "That takes time, a lot of time. And a lot of hard work." Her recognition of and respect for discipline and hard work are evident in her activism and the fact that she enrolled as a mature student in the Fine Arts program at Algoma University in 2005 and graduated with a BFA Honours.

I mention that Canada's national narrative and textbooks do not include any of the problems we've been talking about and need to be rewritten. I know from my reading and discussion with other survivors that it only takes one corrupt administrator to make an institution spiral out of control, which is what happened at Shingwauk and so many other residential schools.

"We know that. And I think Canadians are beginning to know that too. Not through their work, but through ours. When I started here, coming back after spending nine years in the institutions, I had the feeling that I needed to do more, to *do* something about it. Even though I didn't know what was going on, even though I knew little about the history, I felt myself moved in that direction. I followed my instinct. I had no idea of all these stories that were coming forward, no idea what it all meant until I sat down and had a conversation with Don Jackson. Don is my hero, because he helped me to look at it and understand and to realize that there was something that we had to do."

Don Jackson, now retired, was professor and chair of the Department of Law and Politics at Algoma University, a man who knew the history and challenges of the place, a residential school whose reputation had suffered under certain principals, religious blinkers, government parsimony, and neglect.

"So we started by having this reunion, then one interview after another. That's how this whole thing came together."

"You mean the Children of Shingwauk Alumni Association?"

"Yes, it was initially called the Shingwauk Project. Don headed that up in his department. And he used to put money from his own paycheque into that fund. And when I think about that, what a selfless thing to do . . . because he wanted to help. And so we started coming together and talking more and more about what this whole thing was about. And then the stories of sexual abuse hit the fan, so to speak, and opened that chasm. And myself, I was just amazed because I didn't realize while I was here, I hadn't realized what was going on. I didn't find out till much later that some of my friends had been sexually abused. I knew we suffered physical abuse, but to us that was second nature. That's what they did with us. There was no kindness . . . you were pulled out of your loving homes to where there was no kindness."

Shirley speaks of losing her language, not only because of the residential school, but also because her grandfather, an Anglican lay preacher, accepted the party line on assimilation and the superiority of white culture. His position may also have protected Shirley in the residential school, although that's my assumption, not hers.

"When I became a worker in the hospital, why wasn't I as affected as others by all the suffering that accumulates? This troubled me. Then I realized it was because I had learned to live in the moment, not to let it build up and overcome me. You don't think about the past. If you live in the moment nothing can touch you. I was always happy. The Creator made me that way. And like I said, I am an instinctual person."

"You're also a lucky person to have been able to live in the present," I point out. "Many of those who've shared their painful IRS experiences talk about having had to dissociate, close off their emotions, step outside themselves while nasty things were happening. As for erasing painful memories, others had the job done for them by ECT, electro-shock therapy. No anaesthetic, tied down, then the grand mal seizure."

"Yes, that's how a lot of people deal with sexual abuse at a young age. And the hospitals, if they had that kind of equipment to do that, why wouldn't they use it? How depraved. And when I think of it, we were entrusted to the care of those people. I was here when principal Philips was here. He had those really dark and sunken eyes. I felt there was something wrong with that man. Only later did I learn what. We were in a dorm with forty kids in it. And when we talked about that at our meetings years later, one of my friends told me what he did to her. He threatened to send her to a reform school if she talked."

I bring up the subject of the murder of Richard Thomas at Kuper Island Residential School and the travesty of justice it represents, all the way from the school to the police to the coroner.

Shirley downs the last sip of her coffee to control her exasperation, then adds wistfully, "I had a cousin who was in the sanatorium for quite a number of years. Unfortunately, we did not have much contact after I got out of here."

"Fort William?'

"Yes. Recently, President Chamberlain, myself, and Jonathan Dewar met with two ladies from the School of Medicine. They're putting together a meeting of all of those areas of medicine connected with Indigenous patients, so we talked about how we can integrate traditional and conventional medicine. And I think this part that you're talking about—because there's a historic context in the medical arena with regard to Aboriginal people, and how they fared in those hospitals—I think there's a connection here, with a lot of history around it." Shirley pauses to catch her breath. "This needs to be part of that story."

"Some might disagree, because they consider that racism and abuse are all in the past."

"No, no! We live that past daily. Abuse in schools, hospitals, sanatoria, all of it needs to be part of the story."

"How do you fight racism or discrimination?" I ask her. "It's a question that still plagues me, even after three years of interviews."

"You have to be able to mirror it right back at them. The eyes are the mirror of the soul. You need to reflect that racism right back at them, so they feel uncomfortable. I was at the checkout counter recently. There was no greeting. Just the price: $49.78. No please, no thank you, the receipt tossed into the bag. So, I said, 'You know in all the time this transaction has been taking place, you never gave me the time of day. I'm the one who's paying your salary.' I chose not to be angry with the clerk and respond with harsh words. Being angry is a choice. We always have a choice. It takes practice to say to yourself, I want to have a conversation. It's not easy. There was a time I'd get angry. It affected my health. And everyone around me got troubled."

"How did the clerk respond?"

"The next time she was polite."

"A small, but important victory. What about the larger battles?"

"We Missanabie Cree are still trying to get our land back. In 1995, I became chief for ten years. I began to find and bring the people back together. We located 150. Now it's up to four hundred. We're expected to do things with no resources. Twenty-one years later, we've got some land back, but we're still fighting. The government keeps putting up hurdles. I'm not in the Aboriginal Olympics, but I seem to have become an expert at leaping over hurdles."

"How do you keep going?"

"We can't afford to stop now. I keep pouring myself into different areas. I had the opportunity to work from this institution. He's asked me to assemble Shingwauk Elders. My job is to gather them together to talk about how we can bring about change, improve educational opportunities, provide information to non-Indigenous students as well. I was on the board of trustees. We had to fight to keep the old house."

I presume the "he" Shirley refers to is President Chamberlain and that she's talking about the Shingwauk principal's house, a hundred yards east of the library and hall, where I'd talked to Mitch Case the previous day as he made preparations for a feast for Indigenous students.

"It was part of the history, good and bad," Shirley insists, "so I said: 'Let's restore it for something useful.'"

I wonder privately how she feels about the incorporation of Shingwauk Hall into the Algoma campus buildings, but Shirley, reading my thoughts, describes a mature man, a Shingwauk survivor invited to take part in a ceremony at the university, who could not stand being in the building, however altered it was architecturally, and had to leave. These visible reminders of old trauma bring to mind the recent demolition of St. Michael's Residential School in Alert Bay, whose empty shell and dark presence hung over the village for several decades after it closed. It had been put to use by various groups in the community, but never felt right, especially in a community next door to the most highly politicized Indigenous museum I'd ever visited, each recovered artefact accompanied by detailed notes of its significance to the Potlatch ceremony, including when and how it had been confiscated by authorities. Eventually a majority of the people agreed to the building's removal.

When I bring up the Kuper Island Residential School, Shirley interjects: "I know about Kuper. I worked for a while in BC, so I heard about the dumping of the cornerstone into the sea."

The tape and our time together are winding down. As she stands to leave, Shirley gives me a hug and turns at the door to say, "By the way, a few weeks ago, I was appointed Chancellor of Algoma University."

thirty-six

The Road Back East

There are blessings and curses to being on the peripheries of a country the size of Canada. Amongst the blessings, I count the independence and resilience that comes from remoteness, where there is more potential to resist the pressures of homogenization and to develop both individually and collectively. You can see this in the far north, on the east and west coasts, and in some of the less populated areas of the country. The downside is that your opinions and problems are more likely to be ignored. It's notable that most of the discussion of residential schools and issues of Indigenous health and wellbeing seldom focus on the Maritime provinces, and even less on Newfoundland and Labrador. Other than the abuse at Mount Cashell Orphanage in St. John's and the 2013 protest by the Elsipogtog First Nation in New Brunswick against fracking, how often do you read or hear any sustained media coverage of Indigenous issues "down east"?

A welcome exception is a recent article by Stephen Maher in *The National Post* called "Not a Genocide? Ask the Beothuks," in which he responds to Conrad Black's earlier comment in the same newspaper that Indigenous peoples should be grateful for the arrival of Europeans and notes the hostile response this view elicited from First Nations:

> No Beothuks complained. That's because Shanawdithit, the last
> of the Beothuks, died of tuberculosis in Botwood, N.L., on June 6,
> 1829. She was likely not grateful to the Europeans. They drove her

people away from the coast, into the forests and barrens, where the ones who did not starve to death were hunted like animals.[23]

I suppose you could also say that another of the curses of living on the margins is that you might more easily be poisoned or killed with impunity, except that it's been happening to Indigenous peoples in Central Canada as well. Maher compares all these killing fields with what took place during the Spanish Conquest.

Chris Benjamin's book *Indian School Road* is an important contribution to the story of Canada's residential schools and Indigenous health care in the Maritimes. Although he focuses almost exclusively on Shubenacadie Residential School, which opened in Hants, Nova Scotia, in 1930, his book has wider implications for anyone interested in understanding the mindset of the architects and administrators of this deadly educational experiment.

The Mi'kmaq of the Atlantic provinces did not fare well under their colonial masters, though the French had proven more accommodating than the British, whose Governor Edward Cornwallis, installed in 1749, put a bounty on their heads and is said to have paid out £350 for scalps. By 1752, there were only twenty thousand left of an original first-contact population of 200,000; and a century later, their numbers had been reduced to less than a thousand. The remnants—lands stolen, livelihood and spirits damaged—clung to miniscule reserves or lived as beggars on the outskirts of white settlements, mostly around Halifax.

Enlightenment or shame, byproducts of Fabian socialist thought and a re-emergence of Christian evangelism-cum-charity, prompted politicians, priests, and reformers to go to bat for a residential school for the Maritimes, even though the record of such schools had come under severe criticism. D.C. Scott, superintendent of Indian Affairs, who claimed the establishment of Shubenacadie Residential School was one of "the desires of my professional life," had insisted that it be located in clear view of the new railway. This supposed priority and crowning achievement was unwisely located on a sacred Mi'kmaw burial site. It was shoddily built, overcrowded, underfunded, and frequently in the news for mismanagement, negligence, and brutality. The ongoing pattern, Benjamin insists, stems from the fact that "governments still tend to see First Nations as a liability, an expense to be minimized."[24]

Not surprisingly, the testimonies of survivors are often at odds with memory lapses and denial among former teachers in the Sisters of Charity. However, the explosion of sexual abuse lawsuits across Canada in the 1990s against churches and government emboldened those survivors whom fear had long silenced. The struggle for recognition and compensation in Nova Scotia was spearheaded by Nora Bernard, an IRS survivor from Millbrook, Nova Scotia, who rallied lawyers and organized support groups and healing circles that helped shame the government into action. This involved a much-flawed process of compensation that required survivors to prove attendance and describe in excruciating and humiliating detail, more than once, the nature and frequency of physical and sexual abuse.

Canada's long overdue official apology to Indigenous peoples in 2008 has been constantly undercut not only by parsimony, legal intransigence, and a stance of disbelief in what they are being told, but also by public pronouncements from the former government. In addition to saying that the issue of murdered and missing Aboriginal women "is not on our radar," Stephen Harper is on record as saying Canada has no history of colonialism. The former Minister of Aboriginal Affairs Bernard Valcourt tried to diminish the damage of residential schools by calling it "education policy gone wrong." The Gordon Residential School in Saskatchewan was the last to close in 1996, almost ninety years after Peter Bryce described their conditions as criminal, but the systemic racism that fuelled those schools is still with us, as evidenced by substandard housing, polluted water, teen suicide, violence against Indigenous women, and the increasing number of Indigenous men and women in prison and children in foster care.

Benjamin is less concerned with how this ongoing abuse is disguised than in telling us how it can be overcome: "Only when settler Canada can acknowledge its shameful past with open eyes, without excuses and apply the lessons in those mistakes to justice, shedding our 'civilized' sense of superiority, will there be hope for Canada." Topping the list of necessities to achieve this, he says, is ending "the ongoing attempts by our government to control and assimilate Aboriginal peoples."[25]

Although Benjamin does not deal specifically with the question of Indian hospitals in his superb book, there are certainly plenty of references to the illness, brutality, and injuries that sent students to their graves, to sick bays, or to the regional hospitals. He devotes a whole chapter to health care. The medical situation at Schubenacadie was a tragedy of errors. For example, Indian Affairs reminded Father Mackey of his responsibilities and advised him on what amounted to a healthy diet—brown bread, fish, meat, beans—but failed to provide the funds that would make such a diet possible. Dental work was denied, or done on the cheap, without freezing; patients diagnosed with acute TB remained in limbo, not allowed to remain at the school, yet often refused by hospitals or local sanatoria. Outbreaks of flu, syphilis, and diphtheria were not uncommon. Benjamin reports the case of Wayne Nicholas who was so badly treated at the residential school that, when sent to the Truro Hospital with a broken collarbone, he thought he'd gone to heaven, with three square meals a day and affectionate nursing care. Benjamin also writes, at length, of the death of twelve-year-old Josephine Smith who was diagnosed with acute appendicitis. Dr. McInnis recommended she be sent immediately to the nearest hospital, thirty minutes away by car, but Father Mackey decided she could wait until the next day for the train to Halifax, where she died shortly after surgery to remove a gangrenous appendix, her demise officially attributed to pneumonia. Indian Affairs, anxious to avoid any bad publicity, sided with Father Mackey. Dr. McInnis's response says plenty about the value that Indian Affairs placed on Indigenous health: "It is futile to report these cases to the Department as they probably feel as [Mackey] does that they go to Heaven and that it is not worthwhile trying to keep these poor Indian children alive."[26]

In the last five years, I've travelled down Benjamin's Indigenous road by train, plane, car, boat, and books trying to find answers to my own and Joanie Morris's questions about the segregated Indian hospital system and Indigenous health care in general. The experiences people have shared with me about the schools and hospitals have been heartbreakingly similar: hunger, separation anxiety, neglect, brutality, involuntary sterilizations, sexual abuse, shock treatment, and gratuitous drug and surgical experiments, many of which led to permanent disability or death, the causes and burials either falsely recorded or not recorded at all. The government has known about some of these abuses for more than a hundred years, not only from Bryce's report, which the government's own lawyer said left them open to charges of manslaughter, but also from letters of complaint from students and parents that were ignored or scoffed at by bureaucrats at Indian Affairs. But, like the situation at Schubenacadie, nothing was done. The churches, carrying out government policy, added their own special touch: scorn, abuse, threats of hellfire, and hard labour in lieu of education and nurturing.

According to Justin Brake, in an article published in *The Independent.ca* on June 17, 2015, class action suits continue in Newfoundland and Labrador on behalf of residential school students who survived institutions set up before Newfoundland joined Confederation. These survivors were not included in the Official Apology or the federal compensation process. Around one thousand Inuit, Innu, and Mi'kmaq were ignored, their stories of neglect and abuse overshadowed by the revelations from Mount Cashell, where, according to Amelia Reimer, Innu children from Sheshatshiu and other communities were among the victims of sexual abuse.

Brake also quotes Reimer as saying, "People are still being hurt today. Some of it is intergenerational violence; the trauma happened and it gets passed down, and the reactions and the coping skills to this trauma get passed down, whether it be looking for solace in alcohol or substances, whether it be learning to abuse people—domestic violence, child abuse."[27] And, of course, governments delay as long as possible, because foot-dragging is guaranteed to reduce the settlement costs as claimants die off.

Pamela Palmater, a brilliant and articulate Mi'kmaw lawyer and chair of Indigenous Governance at Ryerson University, argues that medical experimentation, not just diseases, claimed lives:

> These children didn't die from smallpox or some other series of unfortunate and unpreventable events in those schools. Nutritional tests and medical experimentations were done on these children only to be denied the benefit of the very medicines created at the expense of their suffering . . . Survivor stories of frequent rapes, forced abortions, and unmarked graves stand in stark contradiction to any notion of a benign education policy. Why else did these schools have graveyards instead of playgrounds?[28]

Palmater goes on to reject the term "cultural genocide" as too easy and convenient for perpetrators, because the term "was specifically left out of the United Nations Convention on the Prevention and Punishment of the Crime of Genocide."[29]

CBC's Mark Quinn quotes Nicky Obed as saying he lost his language, Inuktitut, which alienated him from his home community. He was also sexually abused at the residential schools in St. Anthony, Newfoundland, and Northwest River, Labrador. In the same article, Cindy Dwyer from Nain, Labrador, testifies about being abused and terrified from age five to fifteen by the treatment she received, from beatings and being locked all day in a closet. What she wants is an apology from the International Grenfell Association, who hired the teachers, as well as acknowledgement and compensation from the Canadian government.[30] A few months after these articles appeared, Canada's new Liberal government would address this injustice and offer a belated compensation package.

PART FOUR

RESTORING THE SONG

Lessons for the Hard of Hearing

thirty-seven

Scott Free

Winter rains have turned the lawn to mush, and the picnic table on the deck slowly deteriorates from exposure to the elements. It's cosy enough inside; heat from the glowing chunks of alder and the occasional piece of arbutus in the fireplace insert spreads slowly from room to room. It's one of those days when it feels good to be sitting at my desk writing. Or thinking about writing. I have several Canadian poetry anthologies on my desk, open at the poems of Duncan Campbell Scott.

For me, it seems, writing involves a moral imperative that requires facing the darkest of issues, engaging with them, seeking to understand their origins, and, importantly, critiquing my own position of privilege and power in relation to those issues. I don't consider myself a lugubrious whim-wham indifferent to pain and suffering, but someone who feels lessened by its existence. I carry the injustice and suffering of others around on my back like the dead albatross hanging around the neck of Coleridge's ancient mariner, until I can find a way to understand and give shape to them in my writing. Unlike Coleridge's Ancient Mariner, who killed the albatross and must share the story with every passerby, I may not be to blame for what happened to Indigenous peoples in the distant past, but I enjoy the privileges therefrom and am definitely responsible to see that they are adequately compensated, that remedial action set in motion. And I am certainly accountable for what continues to happen to them as a result of past and present injustices. It has taken me too long to reach this

265

awareness, and my early misreading of poems by the Deputy Superintendent of Indian Affairs is part of the problem.

I discovered Duncan Campbell Scott when I was a graduate student at the University of Toronto. I found his poetry gripping and exotic, and I volunteered to present a seminar paper on the subject. Scott not only noticed Indigenous people, but also wrote about them and—I would learn much later—played a significant role in deciding their fate. Aside from a few lightweight lyrics in the manner of the lesser Romantic poets, Scott had somehow found his way inside the shadowy world of Indigenous culture in Canada and seemed to have tapped a deeper note, a Canadian reality of starvation, violence, and death taking place at the intersection of Indigenous and non-Indigenous cultures. This made his work seem more relevant, more important, and, to my mind, a cut or two above that of his contemporaries. I should say it was the collision—rather than the intersection —of two cultures, one equipped with superior weapons and unbending notions of superiority, progress, and private ownership.

I knew nothing of Scott the bureaucrat and deputy superintendent of Indian Affairs, and was not inclined to seek out that information since the prevailing critical mode of the day was to dismiss biographical detail and consider only the work as it appears on the page. Instead, I saw him as someone in the vanguard of a new and exciting wave of original poetry, fully engaged with what was happening on the ground in Canada, not your typical immigrant poet looking to the motherland with nostalgia. He wrote a ballad about a logger and his lover, both lost while trying to break up a log-jam, thunderous vaulting logs crushing them like a wolf's jaw. In the "The Forsaken," he describes an Indigenous woman who cuts a piece of her own flesh as bait for fish to keep her starving infant alive, and who, as an old woman, is eventually abandoned to the elements by her family, finding rest only in silence and death. "On the Way to the Mission" involves a short narrative of two white villains stalking and eventually shooting an Indigenous trapper, thinking his sled full of furs, only to discover it's the body of his dead wife that he's taking to the mission for spring burial. There's a dignity in these Aboriginal portraits that contrasts with the violence of the interlopers, who are presented as low-life scum, "servants of greed."

The narrative Scott weaves of Canada's original inhabitants is tragic, no question. His Aboriginal subjects are seen as a vanishing race, unable to resist the forces of change. This tragic note touched me deeply, so deeply that I failed to turn a critical eye on the obvious racist assumptions embodied in many of his poems, including a cleverly rhymed sonnet called "The Onondaga Madonna":

> She stands full-throated and with careless pose,
> This woman of a weird and waning race,
> The tragic savage in her face,
> Where all her pagan passion burns and glows;
> Her blood is mingled with her ancient foes,
> And thrills with war and wildness in her veins;
> Her rebel lips are dabbled with the stains
> Of feuds and forays and her father's woes.
>
> And closer in the shawl about her breast,
> The latest promise of her nation's doom,
> Paler than she her baby clings and lies,
> The primal warrior gleaming from his eyes;
> He sulks and burdened with his infant gloom,
> He draws his heavy brows and will not rest.[1]

Along with the barely suppressed eroticism—the careless pose, rebel lips, pagan passion, wildness, and hinted miscegenation—in Scott's depiction of the mother, there is the infant, not trailing innocent clouds of glory like the newborn babe in Wordsworth's "Ode: Intimations of Immortality," but a gloomy, irritable little bundle, possibly a half-breed, and already itching to grow up fast and violent. And, of course, to reinforce the idea of a "weird and waning race" set up in the second line of the sonnet, there is the child's "gloom" that rhymes so tellingly with "doom."

It's embarrassing to have been, as a young academic and would-be poet, so intent on craft that I was blind to this sonnet's underlying racist assumptions. At that point, I had not acknowledged the startling contradictions that could exist in the lives of the writers I admired, the racism of Scott not unlike the anti-Semitism of Ezra Pound. It would be comforting

267

to explain away the racist assumptions of both men as a product of their times if it were not for the fact that such racism is still alive and well in Canada today. Pound, with his radio broadcasts, served as a mouthpiece for the Italian fascists, just as the announcers at Radio Milles Collines stirred up hatred against Tutsis and moderate Hutus during the Rwandan genocide. Scott's poems, however sympathetic on the surface, manage to reinforce the stereotypes of Indigenous peoples as hopeless savages, slaves to their passions and unsavoury traditions, unfit for and unlikely to survive the advent of so-called civilization.

Although Mark Abley reminds us in *Conversations with a Dead Man* that D.C. Scott did not coin or use the phrase "kill the Indian in the child," it is abundantly clear that Scott's policies, if not his personal sentiments, reflected this view and the government's attitude and aims at the highest level. This economic terrorism—keeping *his* Indians starving in order to save money—which amounted to ethnic cleansing, was, of course, a sure way of destroying immune systems and letting sickness, despair, time, and eventually "educators" do the rest.

My struggles to come to terms with the contradictions in Duncan Campbell Scott are not unrelated to my own struggles as a non-Indigenous person to understand and respond to the real history of Canada. And these unfolding truths about our history have been and will continue to be challenging. No one has expressed this challenge better than Paulette Regan in *Unsettling the Settler Within*:

> As a settler ally, I must continuously confront the colonizer-perpetrator in myself, interrogating my own position as a beneficiary of colonial injustice. Exploring the epistemological tensions of working between these two identities means embracing persistent uncertainty and vulnerability. If we have not explored the myths upon which our identity is based, or fully plumbed the depths of our repressed history, we lack a foundation for living in truth. What we have is a foundation of untruths, upon which we have built a discourse of reconciliation that promises to release Indigenous-settler relations from the shackles of colonialism but will actually achieve just the opposite.[2]

Regan's comment is a reminder that racism has many shades, and that my own family was not exempt from employing some of the dubious epithets that can be overheard in those shades. I recall hearing my otherwise generous and accepting father speak of "Jewing" someone down, and spending three of my Saskatchewan years on a farm that had two old work horses, one black and one white, named Nigger and King. My beloved step-grandmother, Carrie Peichl, who wouldn't hurt a fly and was known to feed the occasional Cree family that showed up at our door, could be heard at the supper table telling us to eat all our food and not be like the Indians, whose motto, apparently, was "chicken today, feathers tomorrow." The colonial project requires, and obviously thrives on, its racist agenda, encouraging and tolerating even the most innocuous and unconscious of racist comments.

thirty-eight

Guns, Terms, and Zeal

When my interviews with Elders take me to Yukon, I have the pleasure of spending a couple of hours in the new Kwanlin Dün
Cultural Centre in Whitehorse. As the guide who shows us around pauses
in front of a canoe, I ask her what I will realize seconds later is a stupid
question: do the Indigenous peoples in the North use steam as a means of
bending the wood. Eyebrows raised, and registering a whimsical expres-
sion, she says, "You have to talk to the wood to make it bend."

What a delightful and ironic clock stopper. Perhaps this is what's
beginning to happen now in Canada: the First Nations, Métis, and Inuit
are talking to us and, if we are capable of not just listening but actually
hearing, we are beginning to bend, if only a little. They are also talking to
each other, including those who have become stiff and rigid from centuries of racism and colonial bullying, but have begun to sense the possibility
of transformation in their lives, individually and collectively.

Thinking about the guide's statement, with all its suggestions of intimacy and interrelatedness, leads me to former Crown Attorney Rupert
Ross's *Indigenous Healing*, another of the treasures I acquired during a very
expensive visit to Octopus Books in Ottawa, which has a wonderful selec-
tion of materials by and about Indigenous people. Ross begins with an
instructive epigraph from Hollow Water First Nation in Manitoba: "Much
of what used to be described as 'healing' is now viewed as 'decolonization therapy.'"[3] After a long and impassioned examination of the atrocities

perpetrated on Indigenous peoples, caused by "a host of factors, especially residential schools and racial denigration, over more than a century," Ross concludes that "it no longer matters who intended what result. What does matter is the need to recognize that policies put in place forty or sixty or a hundred years ago remain tragically powerful today and we all have a responsibility to do whatever it takes to get things back on a respectful path again."[4] He addresses throughout his book the matter of "unresolved" or "intergenerational" trauma, which underlies the dysfunction within families and communities and the disproportionate number of Indigenous people in jails.

As an attorney, Ross believes that in the "absence of effective detraumatization or decolonization programs, jails will only do further psychological harm and put communities further at risk. In my view, we should be sending as few people into that environment as we safely can, while helping aboriginal people create rehabilitative programs in both the correctional facilities and the communities themselves. Those programs must recognize the colonial roots of these psychological challenges and offer holistic strategies designed to recover lost psychological ground."[5]

Like Judge John Reilly in Alberta, Crown Attorney Rupert Ross of northern Ontario is appalled to realize how unaware he had been of Indigenous history for most of his life. Growing up next to Indigenous communities, he admits,

> I had no idea whatsoever about how residential schools had touched every aboriginal person I met. It is only in the last half dozen years that I have gained a sense of colonization and the burdens it has imposed on generations of aboriginal people. As a prosecutor, I went north in astounding ignorance, believing that I would serve those communities well simply by prosecuting their criminals and sending them to jail. I had no idea about the people I was encountering or the psychological burdens they carried, primarily from residential school.[6]

Ross was caught in a double-bind as a crown attorney when it came to dealing with extreme cases.

Having watched a couple of generations trying to cope with racism and violence, their anger rendering them a threat to society, Ross despairs at the lack of long-term healing that might have saved them from becoming dangerous offenders. As I had been struggling with the question of Indigenous anger and where it finds release, I was surprised and intrigued by his take on the subject, which struck me initially as insupportable. "In my view," he says, "it is to the immense credit of indigenous people that so few have responded with anger or violence to the intense and pervasive denigration they have suffered for centuries at our hands."[7] I am not so sure about this, especially coming from someone who knows first-hand the frequency of Indigenous encounters with the justice system. To me, this suggests that the anger Ross attributes to abuses suffered in the residential schools, and more than a century of racist and colonial practices, has not disappeared. Rather, it has been turned inward on the self, the family, and the community instead of on the oppressors where it rightly belongs. It seems that, for many, the oppression has been so complete that the usual (i.e., normal) self-protective mechanisms, including what might be called justifiable retaliation, have all been short-circuited.

Kevin Coates, in *#IdleNoMore and the Remaking of Canada*, has a chapter on this subject that seems to agree with Ross but puts a slightly different spin on the question. In a chapter called "The Roots of Aboriginal Anger and Hope," he writes:

> Despite the situation, Aboriginal Canadians are an intensely hopeful people. Even though they have been forced off their lands, marginalized in their home territories, impoverished, controlled by paternalistic governments, and often reviled simply for their "Indianness," they maintain a surprisingly optimistic outlook on their future. Aboriginal people still show up at the negotiating tables. They share their stories, cultures, and ceremonies with continued grace. They seek justice in the Canadian courts and not through acts of violence. Aboriginal communities, even in the midst of their despair and crises, support their Elders, maintain traditions, and protect their traditional lands. The story is not that there have been outbursts from time to time—blockades, protests,

insurrections—but rather that there have been so few of these, and far between. Canadians have spent too little time wondering why Aboriginal people, who suffer such hardships and so many dislocations, have been so non-violent, so rarely disruptive, and so persistent in their pursuit of real solutions. Strong despite the effects of colonialism, determined despite decades of contact and oppression, Aboriginal people remain resilient, determined to claim their rightful place in Canadian society.[8]

Is this hope, or realism coupled with a strong survival instinct? The Gatling gun on loan from the US and used at Duck Lake ended the hope for a Métis homeland in Manitoba. Starvation in Saskatchewan and Alberta brought the great chiefs to their knees on the prairies. Smallpox blankets and contaminated livestock reduced the numbers. And residential schools—that story does not need repeating here. Yet I can't totally dismiss the claims of Ross and Coates.

What I admire about Rupert Ross's book is his willingness to confront his own ignorance, his early racist assumptions, and his unconscious role as a contributor to injustice against Indigenous people. He addresses his doubts, biases, weaknesses, and scepticism about Indigenous concepts and values in a forthright manner, first by weighing Western notions of self and solitude against Indigenous notions of community and belonging. Taking on the Lakota phrase *mitakuya oyasin* ("all my relations"), he begins to reconsider his assumptions about balance and what it means to belong not only to the human community, but also to the community of animate and inanimate things. Coming to terms with the notion of relationship in Indigenous culture, wherein all creation is of a piece—earth, air, water, rocks, trees, animals, people all in relation—he draws important conclusions about the nature of justice:

In short, thinking relationally has drawn me toward a proposition that still sounds strange to me: perhaps the thing that we feel gives us true justice is not really about 'stuff' at all, whether it is the criminal act, the physical loss or injury, the work done or dollars paid in compensation, or even the years served in jail in an attempt to somehow atone for what was done. If our lives are made

273

precious by relationships that nourish us, and if crime is understood as a disruption of those relationships, it may be that justice involves three relational goals: having offenders come to understand, on an emotional level, the relational damage that their crimes have created in others; looking at the relational disharmonies in the offender's life that spawned the crime; and searching for ways to move both parties out of the relational disfigurement that has bound them together in fear, guilt and anger from the moment of the crime.[9]

Although I see greater criminality on the colonial side, the wisdom expressed here reflects what I learned about traditional justice in rural Africa, where the focus is less on retribution and revenge than on restoring balance to the community. Ross pays tribute to this same Indigenous wisdom and honours the creation myths that support it, which foster a view of the universe as a spectacle worthy not of domination and exploitation, but of wonder, respect, and celebration.

It's one thing to talk to the wood, but it is equally important to listen to the wood. In an essay called "Kalhowya Tillicum: Coming Home to the Stories and Songs of the West Coast," author and retired professor Edward Chamberlain reminds us, as Joan Morris and Larry Frolick did earlier, that listening is a necessary art. He quotes poet Robert Bringhurst: "Language listens to the world, I listen with it. What I hear when I listen is a question, which is listening itself."[10] Chamberlain compares a hunter's tracking to reading a text, both of which involve paying attention to the signs, eyes, ears, and other senses on full alert. And he recommends Laurie Ricou's work, *Salal: Listening for the Northwest Understory*, a canny title that conflates world and word, terrain and text, with the implicit suggestion that there are other tribal, regional, and national narratives waiting to be heard beneath the creaking, outdated, false rumblings of the one we've all endured for several centuries, if only we are prepared to listen.

274

thirty-nine

Speaking for Softness_____

A ccording to the World Health Organization definition of 1948, health refers not just to the absence of disease or infirmity, but also "to a state of complete physical, mental and social well-being." If that's so, I don't know many individuals who are healthy for more than brief periods in their lifetime. Even when the body is well-fed and integrated socially, the mind is susceptible to fears, desires, and anxieties that can overwhelm and undermine. Speaking from a relatively comfortable white perspective, Henry David Thoreau observed, "Most men lead lives of quiet desperation and go to the grave with the song still in them." Try to imagine, then, what the word "health" might mean to a young Indigenous woman on a remote reserve, who lives in a mouldy, overcrowded, not properly heated or insulated shack, whose parents, survivors of the residential school, suffer from drug and alcohol addictions and are unable to offer guidance or express affection. Seeing no options in her life, she may turn to drinking, glue-sniffing, or unprotected sex, while images from the intermittently functioning television remind her that life is better "out there" for everyone else, not just because home is off the beaten path, but because, somehow, she is perceived to be of less value than the white population, some of whom are living down the road in better accommodations, with good jobs and salaries and the opportunity of getting out periodically, or permanently.

This situation is the perfect recipe for depression and suicide. Leaving aside the question of genes, good health depends on a lot of variables,

275

including diet, lifestyle, and living conditions in the home, community, and environment. But diet and lifestyle choices (assuming some are available) are affected by the individual's mental health and education. A malnourished child will be a poor learner; a child whose diet lends itself to obesity and diabetes is likely to develop a poor self-image and be handicapped by a weakened immune system. I mention these obvious impediments to good health to indicate that there can be no single solution to what many perceive as a major health crisis amongst Indigenous peoples.

To restore the song that Thoreau says we carry with us even unto the grave requires a broader perspective, a holistic approach that has so far proven impractical or undesirable to governments and the vested interests to which they cater. Such a vision would require seeing life as all-of-a-piece: plants, animals, humans, earth, air, water, all part of a continuum in which destroying or not paying sufficient attention to any one part threatens the rest. This view is incompatible with the boom-and-bust mentality that dominates colonial enterprises and is still rampant in Canada: rape the land, foul the nest, and move on. It's also incompatible with the creation of billionaires. The song, nevertheless, persists; its notes reverberate and its images inspire those beyond the corporate boardrooms and houses of parliament amongst the very people who still have, I must believe, the power to remove and elect governments.

The Brazilian philosopher Paolo Freire, in *The Pedagogy of the Oppressed*, reminds us that written language also has the potential to liberate the oppressed and downtrodden. Once they have words that enable them to name their condition and their oppressors, the oppressed become politicized, capable of throwing off their chains, beginning to fight back and effect change. So education is a significant part of the healing process. Without this, Indigenous anger will continue to be turned inward rather than be directed to the government, a conundrum that brings to mind Jack London's short story "The League of the Old Men," published in 1902. What is so compelling about this story is its acute awareness of the Indigenous perspective on intrusion by white settlers. Imber, the central character in the story, shows up in Dawson City to confess to murdering countless white men, women, and children. In court, preparing to tell his story, he appears to be suffering from "the hopelessness of fatigue and age." When Imber hears his earlier confession being read aloud in court by the young Indigenous translator Howkan, he is amazed and wonders that Howkan can repeat those very words without having heard them spoken. The power of the written word.

As the story proceeds, Imber is asked to explain his actions. He has foreseen the destruction of his people: the wolf hounds, interbreeding with foreign species, become weak; the chief's daughter Noda goes off with a white man, only to return broken and alone with a pale infant under her arm; the young people are seduced into giving up the tribal ways, some of them becoming drunk and disorderly or, like Howkan the translator, scornful of the elders and their traditions. The gift of a pistol in trade results in Koo-So-Tee dying when he tries to kill a grizzly with such a puny weapon. Imber concludes, "And we were bitter, and we said: 'That which for the white man is well, is for us not well. And this be true. There be many white men and fat, but their ways have made us few and lean.'" Trade, Imber explains, has brought disease, increased dependency on the whites, and reduced meat in the forest, and has ushered in famine and dysfunction. The old men of the Whitefish tribe, forced again to become warriors to save their people, decide to eliminate the menace, shooting white foreigners who appear on the river. But the whites keep coming and the old men die off one by one until only Imber is left.

London's story is a strange mixture of ingredients—white racism combined with notions of Indigenous courage and gullibility—but it ends with two men, Imber and the judge, caught up in their respective reveries in the courtroom, leaving the reader to determine the verdict:

> But Imber was dreaming. The square-browed judge likewise dreamed, and all his race rose up before him in a mighty phantasmagoria—his steel-shod, mail-clad race, the lawgiver and the world-maker among the families of men. He saw it dawn red-flickering across the dark forests and sullen seas; he saw it blaze, bloody and red, to full and triumphant noon; and down the shaded slope he saw the blood-red sands dropping into night. And through it all he observed the law, pitiless and potent, ever unswerving and ever ordaining, greater than the motes of men

who fulfilled it or were crushed by it, even as it was greater than he, his heart speaking for softness.[11]

Although there is some small evidence that attitudes and the law are softening, the pace is not fast enough to eliminate the rightful anger of Indigenous peoples in this land. A hollow apology, an occasional victory in court, such as acknowledgement of the Nisga'a rights to their ancestral lands after almost a hundred years of petitions, protests, and legal challenges, and the recent promise of an official inquiry into the missing and murdered Indigenous women and girls, will not address the intergenerational trauma, the poverty and underfunding, the boiled water advisories, the suicides. Some have given up on political solutions, but Taiaiake Alfred, from Kahnawá:ke in the Mohawk Nation and a professor of Indigenous governance at the University of Victoria, rejects this option: "Abstaining from politics is like turning your back on a beast when it is angry and intent on ripping your guts out." Like Imber, he has seen the futility of violence and armed resistance: "a true decolonization movement can emerge only when we shift our politics from articulating grievances to pursuing an organized and political battle for the cause of our freedom."[12]

His book, *Wasáse: Indigenous Pathways of Action and Freedom*, is a different kind of call to arms, a challenge to overcome fear, passivity, and being co-opted by the system. Neither the legal approach, which means allowing your rights to be defined by the state, nor buying into the capitalist economy, as some nations are doing, will bring healing or restore the dignity and freedom that is being crushed by racism and neglect. This is more likely to enrich already well-off tribal councils than to address widespread malaise and unemployment. "To remain true to a struggle conceived within Onkwehonwe values," Alfred asserts, "the end goal of our Wasáse—our warrior's dance—must be formulated as a spiritual revolution, a culturally rooted social movement that transforms the whole of society and a political action that seeks to remake the entire landscape of power and relationship to reflect truly a liberated post-imperial vision."[13] To achieve this, Alfred conceives of a way forward that draws on the discipline and militant non-violence of Buddhism, Mahatma Ghandi's strategy of non-cooperation, and a healthy dose of what he calls anarcho-indigenism.[14]

278
–

His mentors on this path of "non-violent militancy" include Czech playwright and activist Vaclav Havel, North African scholar Albert Memmi, Vietnamese poet-revolutionary Ho Chi Minh, and Frantz Fanon, whose *The Wretched of the Earth*, by laying bare the underlying principles of colonialism, proved to be the gospel for many uprisings throughout the world, including that of the Québécois. Some of the more interesting parts of Alfred's book are the almost Platonic dialogues with two "angry and intelligent" men: Sakej, a Mi'kmaq from Burnt Church and head of the East Coast Warrior Society, and David Dennis, a founder of the West Coast Warrior Society. The task ahead, we learn, involves cultivating political awareness, learning how to channel anger and confront authority, and committing to continuous struggle. Jack London tells us that Imber, too, was dreaming, but does not bother to imagine what that dream might have been. I'd like to think Imber was dreaming of a new kind of man, someone who would take up the struggle guns could not resolve. If so, he was dreaming of Taiaiake Alfred.

I ask my friend Joanie Morris about living in this society as an Indigenous person, and about experiencing racism. She tells me of being repeatedly called a squaw by fellow staff in the hospital where she used to work as a nurse's aid. In her early twenties, she went to a doctor for an internal exam, which turned out to be very painful. When she complained, he said, "Oh come on, you Indian women like it rough." I ask her if this kind of thing still happens forty years later and she describes a recent visit to a female gynaecologist.

"I have cancer, which I take medication for, but it plays havoc with my immune system, so I get frequent bladder and kidney infections. The doctor took one look at my face and she said, 'You need to learn how to wipe yourself.'"

I ask Joanie how she resisted punching the woman in the nose and she explains that she did not want to stoop to the same level, so she turned around and walked out. Add to this the thousands of slights Indigenous children receive at school, the indignities and dangers they can expect to confront as adults in shops, on the job, in the housing market, on the street, and even in cars, where they are likely to be stopped by police, assumed to be drunks, prostitutes, or criminals and viewed with suspicion. Or worse.

Does the settler population have the will and capacity to change its attitudes and behaviour, given the comforts of white privilege, the habit of prejudice, and the pressure from vested interests whose earnings might be affected? I share the perspective of psychologist Carl Jung that maturity is possible, for the individual or the nation, only by acknowledging and coming to terms with the shadow self, the darker side of one's personal and tribal history. That is why I was so persistent in asking survivors of Canada's residential schools and segregated Indian hospitals to go through the painful process of sharing their experiences. A racist society, rather than charging and demoting perpetrators, promotes and rewards a senior military officer who tells his men in Somalia that "the first soldier to shoot a nigger gets a case of champagne"; a racist society makes it possible for a priest to sexually abuse Indigenous children and yet be rewarded with a comfortable retirement in Shaughnessy Heights; and it allows that same individual and his associates to cover up the murder of a boy by telling the police it was a suicide.

This is not the kind of society I want to be part of, but it is one I have to acknowledge and which needs to be changed. I come back to the words of Paolo Freire: "To exist, humanly, is to name the world, to change it. Once named, the world in its turn reappears to the namers as a problem and requires of them a new naming . . . There is no true word that is not at the same time a praxis. Thus, to speak a true word is to transform the world."[15] Praxis is an unusual but important term here, as it refers to words that emanate in action, not just the lip service of an apology, but a course of action that brings about ongoing, substantive change. Canada is changing and needs, if not a new name, at least a revised national narrative, one that embraces change, is capable of compromise, and of speaking truth.

Most Indigenous peoples in Canada have a Transformer figure as part of their mythology, known variously as Qinikalik, Frog, Hare, Raven, or Coyote. Transformer has a sense of humour, which I suppose comes from observing the big picture, and may at times assume the Trickster role, stirring up trouble and turning things upside-down, perhaps for good reason. More often, Transformer moves through the world changing things for the better, causing destructive persons and groups to become positive contributors to society. What would constitute a transformative element in Canada?

While working to improve the living conditions, health, and social opportunities for First Nations, Métis, and Inuit people, we need to think more deeply and critically about our racist assumptions. I believe the Transformer is at work in Canada already, tugging at the blindfolds of many Canadians, allowing us to see what has happened to our Indigenous neighbours and hosts, alerting us to iniquities and inequities in our assumptions and political system. What we do with this hopeful but unsettling awareness will speak volumes about our decency and integrity as a people.

forty

Neighbours, Bridges, and Clams _____

I'm back home now, sitting at my computer trying to process what I've learned, to make as much sense as a I can of the precious hours spent with Indigenous Elders and the painful experiences they've so generously shared with me, sometimes at considerable personal cost. Outside, the heavy winter rains are doing their drum-dance on the metal roof; inside, the dryer spins madly to remove moisture from a load of newly washed clothes. Seasonal winds and tides have resulted in extreme lows and highs, the latter capable of raising the ramp beyond the capacity of its hinges. However, instead of the hinges breaking, the float supporting the ramp sinks a few inches deeper in the water at one end. It's called accommodation, a useful capacity to have. Tonight, though, the tide has ebbed and the sky is so overcast that the dark is absolute. My writing has proceeded by limps and leaps, but a strange sense of balance prevails. I feel humbled by my own ignorance and limitations as a researcher and writer, but I think I'm a little closer to understanding the reasons for setting out on this journey, and a good deal richer for embarking on it and finding some of the guides I needed.

I can't see the sandbars or neighbouring Penelakut Island that was once, geologically speaking, the twin of Thetis. Weeds and shrubs have long since taken over the ground where the Kuper Island Residential School once stood, but its survivors and the community still bear the scars of that experience. I meet folks from Penelakut regularly on the ferry, chat with them, and exchange funny faces with their kids. I don't know why I've resisted talking to more of them about the residential school and the Nanaimo Indian Hospital. Perhaps the experiences of Joan Morris, Belvie Brebber, and those featured in the film *Return to the Healing Circle* have taught me enough. Sometimes important stories and observations come from sources we least expect. Take this one, for instance, which says a lot about residential schools, Penelakut and Indigenous humour and resilience. This comes from Dale Burkholder, a local writer and acute listener with an excellent memory:

> *I worked on the ferry from 1980 to 1985. One of the men I worked with was a native man named Bob Rice. If you look in the local native history, there's lots about the Rice family. Bob was maybe twenty years older than I was. He'd fished commercial for years. He was in his fifties when I met him. I'm not one much for flattery, but I couldn't speak too highly of Bob Rice.*
>
> *He didn't live on the reserve. He lived above the 49th Parallel store in Chemainus and went back and forth in a 14-foot fibreglass, in all weathers. Bob would show up on days when you wondered how the hell he did it. The old hands on the ferry all admitted that he was the best seaman on the boat.*
>
> *Bob was a humble man, but he was solid. He was a deckhand on the ferry, taking orders from the two guys on the bridge, neither of whom were qualified on anything bigger than a rubber duck in a bathtub. He'd just smile. He was always smiling. He had a wicked sense of humour. If the brass were up on the bridge, he would look up at them from the deck and say to me, "Ducks, Dale, can you hear the ducks, farting in shallow water?"*
>
> *He referred to the members of the band who lived on the reserve as "My fellow Canadians." When they tore down the Kuper Island Residential School, he didn't say anything about it. He just watched it, the way he watched everything. On the last day of the shift, we came into the Penelakut dock. The building had been reduced to red brick rubble.*
>
> *Bob said to me, "I went to that school."*

283

*"What was that like?" I asked. He thought about it for a minute.
Then he grinned at me.*

He said, "Holy old blue-eyed snuff-chewing galvanised Christ!"

*That was the only thing he ever said about it. But it stuck with me
somehow. You can use it, if you want to. Bob wouldn't mind.*

A few weeks ago, I listened to an interview on CBC's *The Current* with
Lee Maracle, Drew Hayden Taylor, and Tracy Lindberg talking about the
capacity of Indigenous writing to promote dialogue in Canada and about
the new Minister of Indigenous and Northern Affairs Carolyn Bennett's
suggestion that June be declared Indigenous Book Club Month. Taylor
thought the best Indigenous writing would increase empathy and that
reading Indigenous writers could not help but improve relations. Maracle
suggested the problem went deeper, that Indigenous literature and history needs to be taught early, throughout all levels of the educational
system, to combat racism and ignorance. Tracy, raised in English, wondered if writing in the colonial tongue was, finally, a disservice to her
culture and its own unique language. During this lively discussion, many
subjects, even oral history, came up.[16]

What they had to say echoes the conclusions of Billie Allan and Janet
Smylie in the final paragraph of *First Peoples, Second Class Treatment*:

We end where we began: we as Indigenous peoples must be the
authors of our own stories. It is necessary to interrupting the racism that reduces our humanity, erases our histories, discounts our
health knowledge and practices, and attributes our health disparities and social ills to individual and collective deficits instead of
hundreds of years of violence, marginalization and exclusion.
The stories shared here describe the ways in which racism has
shaped the lives of generations of Indigenous peoples and contributed towards our contemporary health disparities. It is time
for stories of change: change in how we imagine, develop, imple-
ment and evaluate health policies, services and education, change
in how we talk about racism and history in this country. This is
fundamental to shifting what is imagined and understood about
our histories, our ways of knowing and being, our present and our

future, and to ensuring the health and well-being of our peoples for this generation and generations to come.[17]

However important the testimonies and books are, and however much reconciliation appears a desirable goal, these will not be enough to effect the changes and healing that these authors and Pamela Palmater insist are needed. As I could not arrange a meeting with her, I listened to Palmater's interview with Wab Kinew, done while she was a candidate running to become head of the Assembly of First Nations, and her address to the Idle No More audience at Ryerson University, where she is chair of Indigenous Governance. Her message is clear: colonization against our people is ongoing. "By focussing too much on issues of reconciliation and legislation, we forget about the people suffering on the ground."[18] In other words, the AFN's focus must be broader if it hopes to deal concretely with over-representation in the prisons, child welfare, poverty, contaminated water, inadequate health care, sanitation, and housing.

"There is no such thing as benign neglect," Palmater insists. "Canada's racism is conscious, overt and lethal . . . Racism is killing our people and we have to stop it." In her efforts to empower the grassroots, she pulls no punches, listing Canada's two main policy objectives: acquiring Indigenous land and resources and reducing financial responsibility for those displaced. In the process, she makes an apt and provocative verbal distinction: "I say 'eliminated' because that is the word which best describes government intentions. Most people today use the term 'assimilation,' but to my mind, this word is way too soft to describe the design and impact of government policies on Indigenous peoples in Canada."[19]

Kevin Henry, a Hul'qumi'num artist and student at the University of Northern British Columbia, argues that the obsession with statistics and western medical analyses of Indigenous suicides is wrong-headed, because "all of this ignores the root of the problem: suffering stems from the colonization of North America. Colonization is a health determinant, and we need more Indigenous healing so that Indigenous peoples can find solutions in our own way." Like doctor-healer Gabor Maté, Henry is of the opinion that the grief associated with intergenerational trauma can be passed on genetically: "In fact, scholars point to evidence at the cellular

285

level, where powerful environmental stressors can leave an imprint or 'mark' on epigenome-cellular genetic material that is carried into future generations, with devastating consequences."[20]

While there is much debate around the theories of Maté, the work he does in what is called psychoneuroimmunology—science that not only links, but also insists on the interdependence of mind, body, spirit, and environment —opens some doors for the treatment of Indigenous health problems. The suppressing of the immune system as a result of trauma, pain, and stress is more likely to cause disease than the random exposure to bacteria that are around us much of the time. These traumas and stresses, which Maté suggests are often chronic, tend, like Clifford Cardinal's SV40, to undermine or overcome the natural disease suppressors in the immune system.

Maté talks about the deep shame that underlies addictions, the kind found often among abused children, who are told they are evil or worthless and that is why bad things are happening to them. It's this unconscious mind that is behind many of the teen suicides amongst Indigenous youth, who carry the weight of intergenerational trauma, abuse, and lack of love, emanating in self-hatred and shame, the very masks of shame my dear friend Songhees Elder Joanie Morris has been so intent on eliminating. That is what Kevin Henry seeks to address in his appeal to decolonize society and our attitudes to Indigenous health and wellbeing:

> There's a dire need to rebuild health sovereignty for all Indigenous peoples. This means in their own way through their own lens, which will help establish strong foundations for a pedagogy of traditional healing. In any Indigenous community I have visited, decolonization relies on rebuilding language, following in the footsteps of our ancestors, and respecting the natural environment around us. To live is largely seen in Indigenous communities as working to bring back a holistic balance to our societies and be properly actualized in the way of our ancestors, respectfully.[21]

These are some of the incredible guides I've found along the way. Gabor Maté's comments about the link between shame and addiction take me back to the beginning of this journey, when I first met Songhees Elder Joan Morris. I listened to her speak at the TRC hearings in Victoria, then watched her being interviewed on the Nanaimo Daily News Channel, where she explained that fear was the dominant emotion during her experience in the Nanaimo Indian Hospital: "What are they going to do to me next?" I could feel the power in her words and facial expressions caught on tape: "Because you're demeaned, you feel ashamed. So, add that on top of what they do to you, you haven't got much left to fight with, so then the mistrust comes in." Joan, like so many of those her struggle has given me the privilege to meet, has somehow conquered shame and found the stuff she needs for the fight.[22]

In Troy Suzuki's documentary, filmed near Dawson City, ice breaks up on the Yukon River, a violent, cataclysmic affair, huge chunks the size of druidic slabs at Stonehenge turning end over end in their race to summer and the Bering Sea. Franz Kafka insisted that art—writing, music, painting, dance—are capable of shattering the frozen sea within us. That is what's happening here, a rewriting of the national narrative, a breaking of the cultural and political ice. I was reminded of those dramatic images in Troy's film as I made the rounds of the Art Gallery of Alberta in Edmonton, which was hosting an exhibition of paintings by the Indigenous Seven. In Jackson Beardy's work, *Nanabush Catches the Eagle*, Nanabush, the Creator-Transformer, curls up in the belly of a swimming moose, so he can snatch the low-flying eagle from the sky. Nearby, Carl Ray's stunning *Medicine Bear* confirms the interconnectedness of all things, a thin umbilical membrane, a rope of words emerging from its mouth, links bear, turtle, fish, and an indeterminate creature to the embryonic form of a human child. No placid landscapes or still-lifes here; instead, each image is a highly stylized explosion of conflict, colour, and idea, summed up by Beardy's words in large type on the gallery wall: "I no longer see myself torn between worlds but rather as a lifeline between them."

The tide is out. Were it not pitch black, I could walk across the tidal flat to Penelakut, following the tracks of deer and other small animals, creatures who know no borders or boundaries. I hear the low drone of an engine. When I look out the window, moving pinpricks of light penetrate the darkness. It's January, mid-winter, but even without the advantage of sight I recognize the significance of what seems like the dance of fireflies. A few dozen diggers, taking advantage of the extreme low tide, are gathering clams, as if ten thousand years had not passed, the difference being gumboots, jeans, baseball caps, aluminum skiff, and battery-operated headlamps instead of traditional garb and a cedar canoe. The feeling of continuity is comforting, even beautiful, but it's not the image with which to end here when there's so much work to be done and when I know the high level of poverty on Penelakut. Will the new government fulfil its many promises, including the recommendations of the Truth and Reconciliation Commission? I prefer to think of Joan Morris, her health precarious, at a protest rally in Victoria speaking out against racism and environmental degradation, talking to high school students about the seg-regated Indian hospitals, and her excitement at being recently asked to assist in a research project at the University of Victoria; Cree-Lakota *kookum* Lorraine Yuzicapi teaching hundreds of children, youths, and adults about traditional foods and medicines at Treaty 4 gatherings in Saskatchewan; Cree healer Clifford Cardinal searching for the truth about health issues at Goodfish Lake; Mohawk Taiaiake Alfred fine-tuning the strategy in his blueprint for the road ahead; and Mi'kmaw warrior-leader Pam Palmater in downtown Toronto delivering yet another rousing speech, offering that crucial reminder: "We First Nations have been subsidizing the wealth and prosperity and progress of Canadians from our lands and resources . . . And that's the reality that most people don't understand."[23]

I've worked through the night and the first light of dawn has gilded the tips of the firs and cedars on Penelakut. Right on cue, a blood-curdling, pre-historic squawk rends the silence of the morning on Canoe Pass. From my window, I witness an eagle attacking a blue heron on the nearest sandbar. Somehow, amidst the cacophony and flurry of wings, the heron shakes off the deadly talons and begins a slow, upward spiral. "Turning and turning in the widening gyre"—the phrase from a poem by W.B. Yeats comes imme-diately to mind. The blue heron's success seems likely to be short-lived, given the strength and velocity of its attacker. But I'm wrong, as usual. I watch spellbound as the heron's graceful, circular ascent outsmarts and outflanks its assailant, whose speed and ferocity, so deadly on a horizontal or downward angle of attack, lack velocity and manoeuvrability on the lift-off. At an altitude of several hundred feet, the eagle, with a downward dip of the wings, acknowledges its own limitations. It's time for me to do the same.

Notes

INTRODUCTION

1.   Andrea Nanetti and Siew Ann Cheong, "The World as Seen from Venice (1205–1533): As a Case Study of Scalable Web-Based Automatic Narratives for Interactive Global Histories," *Asian Review of World Histories* 4:1 (January 2016), 10.
2.   Charles G.D. Roberts, *In Divers Tones* (1886), (reprint, n.p.: Read Books, 2016).
3.   Earle Birney, "Can. Lit.," in Milton Wilson (ed.), *Poetry of Mid-Century 1940–1960* (Toronto: McClelland and Stewart, 1964), 37.
4.   David Ljunggren, "Every G20 Nation Wants to Be Canada, Insists PM," *Reuters*, September 25, 2009, http://www.reuters.com/article/columns-us-g20-canada-advantages-idUSTRE58P05Z20090926.
5.   Herschel Hardin, *A Nation Unaware: The Canadian Economic Culture* (Vancouver: J.J. Douglas, 1974), 20.

PART ONE—JOANIE'S PEOPLE

1.   Ernie Crey and Suzanne Fournier, *Stolen from Our Embrace: The Abduction of First Nations Children and the Restoration of Aboriginal Communities* (Vancouver: Douglas & McIntyre, 1997), 61.
2.   Ibid., 72.
3.   John Milloy, *A National Crime: The Canadian Government and the Residential School System 1879 to 1986* (Winnipeg: University of Manitoba Press, 1999), 121.
4.   Canada, Royal Commission on Aboriginal Peoples, *Report of the Royal Commission on Aboriginal Peoples*, vol. 1: *Looking Forward, Looking Back* (Ottawa: The Commission, 1996), 334.
5.   Milloy, *A National Crime*.
6.   Thomas B. Berger, *A Long and Terrible Shadow: White Values, Native Rights in the Americas since 1492* (Vancouver: Douglas & McIntyre, 1991), 28–29. Using figures based on a population of 25 million in Mexico, dwindling to 750,000 by the early seventeenth century, Berger calculates that only 3 per cent survived.

7. Laurie Meijer Drees, *Healing Histories: Stories from Canada's Indian Hospitals* (Edmonton: University of Alberta Press, 2013), 179–180.

8. Ian Mosby, "Administering Colonial Science: Nutrition Research and Human Biomedical Experimentation in Aboriginal Communities and Residential Schools, 1942–1952," *Social History* 46, no. 91 (May 2013): 148.

9. Mosby, "Administering Colonial Science," 147.

10. Ibid., 148.

11. Mary-Ellen Kelm, *Colonizing Bodies: Aboriginal Health and Healing in British Columbia, 1900–50* (Vancouver: UBC Press, 1998), xix.

12. Michael Harkin, "Contested Bodies: Affliction and Power in Heiltsuk Culture and History," *American Ethnologist* 21, no. 3 (1994): 589.

13. Cited by Francis Parkman, *The Conspiracy of Pontiac and the Indian War after the Conquest of Canada*, 6th ed. (Boston: Little, Brown, 1886), vol. 2, p. 39. Posted on Peter d'Errico's webpage, http://www.umass.edu/legal/derrico/amherst/lord_jeff.html.

14. From the journal of William Trent, in John W. Harpster, *Crossroads: Descriptions of Western Pennsylvania 1720–1829* (Pittsburgh: University of Pittsburgh Press, 1986 (1938), 103.

15. Peter Bryce, *The Story of a National Crime: Being an Appeal for Justice to the Indians of Canada* (Ottawa: James Hope & Sons, 1922), 4.

16. Meijer Drees, *Healing Histories*, n.p.

17. Pat Sandiford Grygier, *A Long Way from Home: The Tuberculosis Epidemic Among the Inuit* (Kingston: McGill-Queen's University Press, 1994), 176.

18. Ibid., 97–98.

19. Ibid., 123.

20. Peter Grant, "An Interview with Colin Brown," *Pacific Rim Review of Books*, 11, http://www.prrb.ca/articles/issue11-grant.htm.

21. Ibid.

PART TWO—HEARTLAND

1. Nancy Thompson, "Watson Lake Families Seek Answers from Yukon Hospital Corp," CBC Radio (North), November 26, 2013, cbc.ca/news/canada/north/watson-lake-families-seek-answers-from-yukon-hospital-corp-1.2440058.

2. Dara Culhane Speck, *An Error in Judgement: The Politics of Medical Care in an Indian/White Community* (Vancouver: Talonbooks, 1987).

3. David Laird, J.H. Ross, and J.A.J. McKenna, Report of Indian Treaty Commissioners for Treaty No. 8. Winnipeg, MA, 22 September 1899, https://www.aadnc-aandc.gc.ca/eng/1100100028813/1100100028853.

4. Ibid.

5. Charles Camsell Hospital History Committee, *The Camsell Mosaic: The Charles Camsell Hospital, 1945–1985* (Edmonton: Charles Camsell Hospital History Committee, 1985), n.p.

6. Ibid.

7. Meijer Drees, *Healing Histories*, n.p.

8. Maureen K. Lux, *Medicine That Walks: Disease, Medicine and Canadian Plains Native People, 1880–1940* (Toronto: University of Toronto Press, 2001), 38.

9. *Official Debates of the House of Commons of the Dominion of Canada*, 4th Session, 4th Parliament, vol. 12 (1882) (Ottawa: Maclean, Roger & Co., 1882), 1186.

10. Department of Indian Affairs, Superintendent D.C. Scott to Indian Agent General Major D. McKay, DIA Archives, RG 1- Series, 12 April 1910.

11. Department of Indian Affairs, "Correspondence relating to tuberculous among the Indians in the various agencies across Canada 1908–1910," File 140, 754-1, cited in Lux, *Medicine That Walks*, 132.

12. Lux, *Medicine That Walks*, 4.

13. Ibid., 222.

14. Harold Cardinal, *The Unjust Society: The Tragedy of Canada's Indians* (Edmonton: M.G. Hurtig, 1969), 145.

15. *Statutes of the Province of Alberta 1928 Passed in the 2nd Session of the 6th Legislative Assembly*, "The Sexual Sterilization Act," (Edmonton: King's Printer, 1928), 117, http://ourfutureourpast.ca/law/page.aspx?id=2906151.

16. Karen Stote, *An Act of Genocide: Colonization and the Sterilization of Aboriginal Women* (Black Point, NS: Fernwood Publishing, 2015), n.p.

17. Betty Ann Adam, "Saskatchewan Women Pressured to Have Tubal Ligations," *Saskatoon Star Phoenix*, November 17, 2015.

18. Cardinal, *The Unjust Society*, n.p.

19. Ibid., n.p.

20. Ibid., n.p.

21. Ibid., n.p.

22. Ibid., n.p.

23. Candace Savage, *A Geography of Blood: Unearthing Memory from a Prairie Landscape* (Vancouver: Greystone Books, 2012), 62.

24. Ibid., 111.

25. Ibid., n.p.

26. Margaret Atwood, *Survival: A Thematic Guide to Canadian Literature* (Toronto: House of Anansi Press, 1972), 112.

27. http://www.sv40foundation.org.

28. Debbie Bookchin and James Schumacher, *The Virus and the Vaccine: Contaminated Vaccine, Deadly Cancers and Government Neglect* (New York: St. Martin's Griffin, 2004), n.p.

29. *Time Magazine*, n.d, n.p.

30. Marcia Angell, "Medical Research: The Dangers to the Human Subject," *New York Review of Books*, November 19, 2015, http://www.nybooks.com/articles/2015/11/19/medical-research-dangers-human-subjects/.

31. Bookchin and Schumacher, *The Virus and the Vaccine*, n.p.

32. Ibid., n.p.

33. Cited in Ibid., chapter 14.

34. Bookchin and Schumacher, *The Virus and the Vaccine*, chapter 14.

35. James Daschuk, *Clearing the Plains: Disease, Politics of Starvation and the Loss of Aboriginal Life* (Regina: University of Regina Press, 2013), ix.

36. Ibid., x.

37. Ibid., x.

38. Ibid., xv.

39. Ibid., xix.

40. Ibid., xix.

41. Ibid., xxi.

42. Ibid., 123.

43. Ibid., 118; Lux, *Medicine That Walks*, 38.

44. Allan and Smylie, *First Peoples, Second Class Treatment: The Role of Racism in the Health and Well-being of Indigenous Peoples in Canada* (Toronto: Wellesley Institute, St. Michael's Hospital, 2015), 19.

45. Ibid., 19.

46. Ibid., 23.

47. Ibid., 43.

48. http://ncsaca.harmonyapp.com/programs/corrections/buffalo-sage-wellness-house/.

49. Kevin Johnson, "'Toughness on Crime Gives Way to Fairness, Cost Reality," *USA Today*, March 30, 2014.

50. Criminal Code (R.S.C., 1985, c. C-46), available at http://laws-lois.justice.gc.ca/eng/acts/C-46/page-180.html#h-264, also cited in Reilly, *Bad Medicine: A Judge's Struggle for Justice in a First Nations Community* (Victoria: Rocky Mountain Books, 2010), 221–222.

51. Government of Canada, "Restorative Justice—A Worthy Approach," Correctional Service Canada, http://www.csc-scc.gc.ca/restorative-justice/003005-0007-eng.shtml.

52. Deskaheh, "The Last Speech of Deskaheh" (1917), *Indymedia*, http://rochester.indymedia.org/node/878.

53. Nancy J. Turner and Katherine L. Turner, "Where Our Women Used to Get the Food: Cumulative Effects and Loss of Ethnobotanical Knowledge and Practice; Case Study from Coastal British Columbia," *Botany* 86, no. 2 (2008): 105.

54. Ibid., 109.

55. Ibid., 113.

56. Larissa Burnouf, "Horrific Abuse Accompanied TB Treatment," *Eagle Feather News* 16, no. 8 (August 2013): 12.

57. Maureen K. Lux, *Separate Beds: A History of Indian Hospitals in Canada, 1920s–1980s* (Toronto: University of Toronto Press, 2016), 209–210.

58. Burnouf, "Horrific Abuse Accompanied TB Treatment," 12.

59. Richard Wagamese, "Witholding Stories Denies the Truths," *Eagle Feather News* 16, no. 8 (August 2013): 16.

60. Catherine Mitchell, "Perspective: 57 Years of Silence," *Winnipeg Free Press*, December 4, 2009, http://www.winnipegfreepress.com/local/57-years-of-silence-42868487.html.

61. Verna Kirkness, in Celia Haig-Brown, *Resistance and Renewal: Surviving the Indian Residential School* (Vancouver: Arsenal Press, 1998), 141.

62. Patricia Monture-Angus, *Thunder in My Soul: A Mohawk Woman Speaks* (Black Point, NS: Fernwood Publishing, 1995), 100.

63. Alan Cairns, *First Nations and the Canadian State: In Search of Coexistence*, 2002 Kenneth MacGregor Lecturer (Kingston, ON: The Institute of Intergovernmental Relations, Queen's University, 2005), 2.

64. Heather Robertson, *Reservations Are for Indians* (Toronto: J. Lewis & Samuel, 1970), xiv.

65. Ibid., 55–56.

66. Ibid., 58.

67. Ibid., 83.

68. Ibid., 84.

69. Ibid., 109.

70. Ibid., 117.

71. Ibid., 131.

72. Tisdall, in Ibid., 133–138.

73. Ibid., 143.

74. Ibid., 172.

75. Ibid., 275–276.

76. Billie Allan and Janet Smylie, *First Peoples, Second Class Treatment: The Role of Racism in the Health and Well-being of Indigenous Peoples in Canada* (Toronto: Wellesley Institute, St. Michael's Hospital, 2015), 19.

77. Leslie McCartney, "Respecting First Nations Oral Histories: Copyright Complexities and Archiving Aboriginal Stories," in Annis May Timpson (ed.), *Thoughts: The Impact of Indigenous Thought in Canada* (Vancouver: UBC Press, 2009), 78.

78. Ibid., 89.

79. S.D. Gaudin, *Forty-four Years with the Northern Crees* (Toronto: Mundy-Goodfellow, 1942), n.p. Available at http://www.ourroots.ca/toc.aspx?id=8161&qryID=7bfd9d85-468f-45d9-be02-6fbcad7ef956.

80. Ibid.

81. Ibid.

82. Velvet Maud, "Understanding Narratives of Illness and Contagion as a Strategy to Prevent Tuberculosis among Métis in Southern Manitoba," MA thesis (University of Saskatchewan, 2012), 39.

83. Julie Cruikshank, "Oral Tradition and Oral History: Reviewing Some Issues," *The Canadian Historical Review* 75, no. 3 (September 1994): 403–418.

84. Ibid.

85. Margaret Atwood, *Two-Headed Poems* (Toronto: Oxford University Press, 1978), 75.

86. Hugh Brody, *Maps and Dreams* (New York: Pantheon Books, 1981), 274.

87. Claude Lévi-Strauss, "A Writing Lesson," *Tristes tropiques* (New York: Criterion, 1961), 292.

88. Thomas Berger, *A Long and Terrible Shadow: White Values, Native Rights in the Americas Since 1492* (Vancouver: Douglas & McIntyre, 1991), 150.

89. Quoted in Ibid., 153.

90. Grand Council Treaty #3, "Submission to the Ipperwash Inquiry," *The Ipperwash Inquiry, The Honourable Sidney B. Linden, Commissioner*, May 31, 2007, https://www.attorneygeneral.jus.gov.on.ca/inquiries/ipperwash/policy_part/projects/pdf/Chiefs_of_Ontario-Grand_Council_Treaty_3.pdf.

91. Ibid.

92. Theodore Fontaine, *Broken Circle: The Dark Legacy of Indian Residential Schools, A Memoir* (Victoria: Heritage House, 2010), 125.

93. "One on One: Charlie Angus and James Daschuk" (Regina: Reality Publishing, University of Regina Press TV, 2013), https://youtu.be/gW7js37zK7Q.

94. James Daschuk, "When Canada Used Hunger to Clear the West," *Globe and Mail*, July 19, 2013.

95. Lux, *Medicine That Walks*, 15–16.

96. Ibid., 38.

97. Ibid., 45.

98. Ibid., 110.

99. Ibid., 140.
100. Ibid., 213.
101. Fontaine, *Broken Circle*, 233–234.
102. Ibid., 173.

PART THREE—THE LONG SENTENCE

1. Ryan McMahon, "Red Man Laughing: The Wab Kinew Interview," *The Red Man Laughing Podcast*, Season 5, October 30, 2015, https://www.redmanlaughing.com/listen/2015/10/red-man-laughing-the-wab-kinew-interview.

2. George Hutchison and Dick Wallace, *Grassy Narrows* (Toronto: Van Nostrand Reinhold, 1977), 174.

3. Anastasia M. Shkilnyk, *A Poison Stronger than Love: The Destruction of an Ojibwa Community* (New Haven: Yale University Press, 1985), 16.

4. Amnesty International, "Grassy Narrows: Provincial Inaction on Mercury Contamination Inexcusable," *Human Rights Now* (Amnesty Canada blog), June 18, 2015, http://www.amnesty.ca/blog/grassy-narrows-provincial-inaction-on-mercury-contamination-inexcusable.

5. Jody Porter, "Ear Experiments Done on Kids at Kenora Residential School," *CBC News*, August 8, 2013, http://www.cbc.ca/news/canada/thunder-bay/ear-experiments-done-on-kids-at-kenora-residential-school-1.1343992.

6. Ian Adams, "The Lonely Death of Charlie Wenjack," *Maclean's Magazine*, http://www.macleans.ca/society/the-lonely-death-of-chanie-wenjack/ [full citation to come].

7. Hugh Hazelton, *Latinocanadá: A Critical Study of Ten Latin American Writers of Canada* (Montreal: McGill-Queen's University Press, 2007), n.p.

8. David Wu, "An Interview with Elder Fred John, Part 1," *Caring for Our Children* (newsletter), *BC Aboriginal Care Society* 13, no. 5 (Jan-Feb 2011), p. 1, http://www.acc-society.bc.ca/files_new/documents/CFOCJan-Feb11Final.pdf .

9. Ibid., 2.

10. Klisala Harrison, "'Singing My Spirit of Identity': Aboriginal Music for Well-being in a Canadian Inner City," *MUSIcultures* 36 (2009), 5.

11. Quoted in John Ackerman, *Dylan Thomas: His Life and Work* (London: Macmillan, 1996), 53.

12. Yvonne Boyer, *Moving Aboriginal Health Forward: Discarding Canada's Legal Barriers* (Saskatoon: Purich, 2014), n.p.

13. Ibid., n.p.

14. Ibid., n.p.

15. Brandon University, "Canada Research Chair in Aboriginal Health and Wellness Comments on Racism in Health Care" (news webpage), *Brandon University*, March 2, 2015, https://www.brandonu.ca/news/2015/03/02/crc-aboriginal-health-wellness-racism-health-care/.

16. Albert Dumont, *Of Trees and Their Wisdom: Poetry and Short Stories* (Ottawa: Turtle Moons Press, 2009), n.p.

17. Amanda Goldrick-Jones and Herbert Rosengarten (eds.), *The Broadview Anthology of Poetry* (Peterborough: Broadview Press, 1993), 628.

18. Earle Birney, *The Essential Earle Birney*, ed. by Jim Johnstone (Erin, ON: The Porcupine's Quill, 2014), 28.

19. Malcolm Mackenzie Ross, *The Impossible Sum of Our Traditions: Reflections on Canadian Literature* (Vancouver: McClelland & Stewart, 1986), 193.

20. Joseph Boyden, *Three Day Road* (Toronto: Penguin Canada, 2008), Chapter 20.

21. Milan Kundera, *The Book of Laughter and Forgetting: A Novel* (New York: Knopf, 1980), n.p.

22. J.R. Miller, *Shingwauk's Vision: A History of Native Residential Schools* (Toronto: University of Toronto Press, 1996), 9.

23. Stephen Maher, "Not Genocide? Ask the Beothuks," *The National Post*, June 11, 2005, http://news.nationalpost.com/full-comment/stephen-maher-not-genocide-ask-the-beothuks.

24. Chris Benjamin, *Indian School Road: Legacies of the Shubenacadie Residential School* (Halifax: Nimbus, 2014), n.p.

25. Ibid., n.p.

26. Ibid., 54–60.

27. Reimer, in Justin Brake, "No Reconciliation for N.L. Residential School Survivors, Yet," *The Independent*, June 19, 2015, http://theindependent.ca/2015/06/19/no-reconciliation-for-n-l-residential-school-survivors-yet/.The Independent.ca on June 17, 2015.

28. Pamela Palmater, "Canadian and Church Officials Must Be Held Accountable for Genocide," *telesurtv*, June 17, 2015, http://www.telesurtv.net/english/opinion/Canadian-and-Church-Officials-Must-be-Accountable-for-Genocide-20150617-0033.html.

29. Ibid.

30. Mark Quinn, "Residential School Students Still Want Apology, Compensation," *CBC News*, September 28, 2015, http://www.cbc.ca/news/canada/newfoundland-labrador/residential-school-students-still-want-apology-compensation-1.3245841.

PART FOUR—RESTORING THE SONG

1. Malcom Mackenzie Ross (ed.), *Poets of the Confederation: Duncan Campbell Scott, Archibald Lampman, Bliss Carman, Charles G.D. Roberts* (Toronto: McClelland & Stewart, 1960), 90.

2. Paulette Regan, *Unsettling the Settler Within: Indian Residential Schools, Truth Telling, and Reconciliation in Canada* (Vancouver: UBC Press, 2010), 236.

3. Rupert Ross, *Indigenous Healing: Exploring Traditional Paths* (Toronto: Penguin, 2014), 185.

4. Ibid., 179.

5. Ibid., 177.

6. Ibid., 154.

7. Ibid., 63.

8. Kevin Coates, *#IdleNoMore and the Remaking of Canada* (Regina: University of Regina Press, 2015), 23–24.

9. Ross, *Indigenous Healing*, 20–21.

10. Quoted in J. Edward Chamberlain, "*Klahowya Tillicum*: Coming Home to the Songs and Stories of the West Coast," *Journal of Canadian Studies* 46, no. 2 (Spring 2012): 99–121.

11. Jack London, "The League of Old Men," in Gary Geddes (ed.), *Skookum Wawa: Writings of the Canadian Northwest* (Toronto: Oxford University Press, 1975), 181ff.

12. Taiaiake Alfred, *Wasáse: Indigenous Pathways of Action and Freedom* (Peterborough: Orchard Park, 2009), 20, 22.

13. Alfred, *Wasáse*, 27.

14. Ibid., 45.

15. Paulo Freire, *Pedagogy of the Oppressed* (New York: Continuum, 2000), 76, 75.

16. "First Nations Authors Discuss Carolyn Bennett's Indigenous Book Club Month," by Connie Walker, *The Current*, CBC, January 8, 2016.

17. Allan and Smylie, *First Peoples, Second Class Treatment*, 44.

18. Wab Kinew, "Interview with Pam Palmater—Candidate for AFN National Chief," *NetNewsLedger*, posted June 27, 2012, http://www.netnewsledger.com/2012/06/27/interview-pam-palmater-candidate-afn-nationa-chief/.

19. Pamela Palmater, *Indigenous Nationhood: Empowering Grassroots Citizens* (Black Point, NS: Fernwood Publishing, 2015), 5, 56.

20. Kevin Henry, "Colonialism Is a Public Health Problem," May 3, 2016, https://ricochet.media/en/1140/colonialism-is-a-public-health-problem.

21. Ibid.

22. "Nanaimo Indian Hospital," interview with Joan Morris, *Nanaimo Daily News*, uploaded December 15, 2011, to NanaimoDailyNews channel, https://youtu.be/ZUOuUo79zU8.

23. "Idle No More: Indigenous-Led Protests Sweep Canada for Native Sovereignty and Environmental Justice," by Amy Goodman, Democracynow.org, December 26, 2012, https://www.democracynow.org/2012/12/26/idle_no_more_indigenous_led_protests.

Bibliography

Abley, Mark. *Conversations with a Dead Man: The Legacy of Duncan Campbell Scott.* Madeira Park: Douglas & McIntyre, 2013.

Ackerman, John. *Dylan Thomas: His Life and Work.* London: Macmillan, 1996.

Adam, Betty Ann. "Saskatchewan Women Pressured to Have Tubal Ligations." *Saskatoon Star Phoenix.* November 17, 2015.

Adams, Howard. *Prison of Grass: Canada from a Native Point of View.* Saskatoon: Fifth House, 1989.

Adams, Ian. "The Lonely Death of Charlie Wenjack." *Macleans Magazine.* February 1, 1967, 30–31, 38–39, 42–44, 49.

Alfred, Agnes. *Paddling to Where I Stand.* Ed. by Martine J. Reid. Trans. by Daisy Sewid-Smith. Vancouver: UBC Press, 2004.

Alfred, Taiaiake. *Wasáse: Indigenous Pathways of Action and Freedom.* Peterborough: Orchard Park, 2009.

Allan, Billie, and Janet Smylie. *First Peoples, Second Class Treatment: The Role of Racism in the Health and Well-being of Indigenous Peoples in Canada.* Toronto: Wellesley Institute, St. Michael's Hospital, 2015.

Amnesty International. "Grassy Narrows: Provincial Inaction on Mercury Contamination Inexcusable." *Human Rights Now* (Amnesty Canada blog), June 18, 2015, http://www.amnesty.ca/blog/grassy-narrows-provincial-inaction-on-mercury-contamination-inexcusable.

Angell, Marcia. "Medical Research: The Dangers to the Human Subject." *New York Review of Books.* November 19, 2015.

Angus, Charlie. *Children of the Broken Treaty: Canada's Lost Promise and One Girl's Dream.* Regina: University of Regina Press, 2015.

Annett, Kevin D. *Hidden from History: The Canadian Holocaust.* Vancouver: Truth Commission into Genocide in Canada, 2001.

Armstrong, Jeannette C. *Slash.* Penticton: Theytus Books, 1985.

Arnett, Chris. *Terror on the Coast: Land Alienation and Colonial War on Vancouver Island and the Gulf Islands, 1849–1863.* Burnaby: Talonbooks, 1999.

Asikinack, William, and Kate Scarborough. *Exploration into North America*. Philadelphia: Chelsea House, 2000.

Asikinack, William, and Kate Scarborough. *North America (Exploring History)*. London, UK: Chrysalis Children's Books, 2003.

Atwood, Margaret. *The Journals of Susanna Moodie*. Toronto: Oxford University Press, 1970.

Atwood, Margaret. *Two-Headed Poems*. Toronto: Oxford University Press, 1978.

Barthes, Roland, Richard Miller, and Richard Howard. *The Pleasures of the Text*. New York: Hill and Wang, 1975.

Beaton, Brian. "2nd Walk for Mother Earth from Grassy Narrows First Nation to Ottawa." *MediaKnet*. September 22, 2009, http://media.knet.ca/node/7317.

Benjamin, Chris. *Indian School Road: Legacies of the Shubenacadie Residential School*. Halifax: Nimbus, 2014.

Berger, John. *And Our Faces, My Heart, Brief As Photos*. New York: Pantheon Books, 1984.

Berger, Thomas B. *A Long and Terrible Shadow: White Values, Native Rights in the Americas Since 1492*. Vancouver: Douglas & McIntyre, 1991.

Birney, Earle. *The Essential Earle Birney*. Ed. by Jim Johnstone. Erin, ON: The Porcupine's Quill, 2014.

Blondin-Perrin, Alice. *My Heart Shook Like a Drum: What I Learned at the Indian Mission School, Northwest Territories*. Ottawa: Borealis Press, 2009.

Bookchin, Debbie, and James Schumacher. *The Virus and the Vaccine: Contaminated Vaccine, Deadly Cancers and Government Neglect*. New York: St. Martin's Griffin, 2004.

Boyden, Joseph. *Three Day Road*. Toronto: Penguin Canada, 2008.

Boyer, Yvonne. *Moving Aboriginal Health Forward: Discarding Canada's Legal Barriers*. Saskatoon: Purich, 2014.

Brake, Justin. "No Reconciliation for N.L. Residential School Survivors, Yet." *The Independent*. June 19, 2015, http://theindependent.ca/2015/06/19/no-reconciliation-for-n-l-residential-school-survivors-yet/.

Brandon University. "Canada Research Chair in Aboriginal Health and Wellness Comments on Racism in Health Care," *Brandon University*, March 2, 2015, https://www.brandonu.ca/news/2015/03/02/crc-aboriginal-health-wellness-racism-health-care/.

Bringhurst, Robert. *The Tree of Meaning: Thirteen Talks*. Kentville: Gaspereau Press, 2006.

Brissenden, Constance, Oskiniko Larry Loyie, and Wayne K. Spears. *Residential Schools: With the Words and Images of Survivors*. Brantford, ON: Indigenous Education Press, 2014.

Brody, Hugh. *Maps and Dreams*. New York: Pantheon Books, 1981.

Brown, Dee. *Bury My Heart at Wounded Knee: An Indian History of the American West*. New York: Holt, Rinehart & Winston, 1971.

Bryce, Peter. *The Story of a National Crime: Being an Appeal for Justice to the Indians of Canada*. Ottawa: James Hope & Sons, 1922.

Burnouf, Larissa. "Horrific Abuse Accompanied TB Treatment." *Eagle Feather News* 16, no. 8 (August 2013): 12.

Cairns, Alan C. *First Nations and the Canadian State: In Search of Coexistence*. 2002 Kenneth MacGregor Lecturer. Kingston, ON: The Institute of Intergovernmental Relations, Queen's University, 2005.

Campbell, Maria. *Halfbreed*. New York: Saturday Review Press, 1973.

Canada, Royal Commission on Aboriginal Peoples. *Report of the Royal Commission on Aboriginal Peoples*, 5 vols. Ottawa: The Commission, 1996.

Cardinal, Harold. *The Unjust Society: The Tragedy of Canada's Indians*. Edmonton: M.G. Hurtig, 1969.

Carr, Paul R., Darren E. Lund, eds., *Revisiting The Great White North? Reframing Whiteness, Privilege, and Identity in Education*. Rotterdam: Sense Publishers, 2015.

Carr, Paul, and Darren E. Lund, eds. *The Great White North? Exploring Whiteness, Privilege, and Identity in Education*. Rotterdam: Sense Publishers, 2007.

Carter, Sarah. *Lost Harvests: Prairie Indian Reserve Farmers and Government Policy*. Montreal: McGill-Queen's University Press, 1993.

Chamberlain, J. Edward. "*Klahowya Tillicum*: Coming Home to the Songs and Stories of the West Coast." *Journal of Canadian Studies*, 46, no. 2 (Spring 2012): 99–121.

Chamberlain, J. Edward. *Living Language and Dead Reckoning: Navigating Oral and Written Traditions*. Vancouver: Ronsdale Press, 2006.

Charles Camsell Hospital History Committee. *The Camsell Mosaic: The Charles Camsell Hospital, 1945–1985*. Edmonton: Charles Camsell Hospital History Committee, 1985.

Clarke, Chris, K'änáchá Group, and Sharon Moore (eds.). *Tr'ëhuhch'in Näwtr'udäh'a (Finding Our Way Home)*. Dawson City, YK: Tr'ondëk Hwëch'in, 2009.

Clements, Marie Humber, and Rita Leistner. *The Edward Curtis Project: A Modern Picture Story*. Vancouver: Talonbooks, 2010.

Coates, Kenneth. *#IdleNoMore and the Remaking of Canada*. Regina: University of Regina Press, 2015.

Crey, Ernie, and Suzanne Fournier. *Stolen from Our Embrace: The Abduction of First Nations Children and the Restoration of Aboriginal Communities*. Vancouver: Douglas & McIntyre, 1997.

Cruikshank, Julie. "Oral Tradition and Oral History: Reviewing Some Issues." *The Canadian Historical Review* 75, no. 3 (September 1994): 403–418.

Cryer, Beryl Mildred, and Chris Arnett. *Two Houses Half-Buried in Sand: Oral Traditions of the Hul'q'umi'num' Coast Salish of Kuper Island and Vancouver Island*. Vancouver: Talonbooks, 2008.

Culhane Speck, Dara. *An Error in Judgement: The Politics of Medical Care in an Indian/White Community*. Vancouver: Talonbooks, 1987.

Cullingham, James, director. *Duncan Campbell Scott: The Poet and the Indians* (film). Tamarack Productions and NFB, 1995.

Dagg, Mel. *The Women on the Bridge*. Saskatoon: Thistledown Press, 1992.

Daschuk, James. *Clearing the Plains: Disease, Politics of Starvation and the Loss of Aboriginal Life*. Regina: University of Regina Press, 2013.

Daschuk, James. "When Canada Used Hunger to Clear the West." *Globe and Mail*, July 19, 2013.

Daschuk, James. "One on One: Charlie Angus and James Daschuk." Regina: Reality Publishing, University of Regina Press TV, 2013. https://youtu.be/gW7js37zK7Q.

Davis, Robert, and Mark Zannis. *The Genocide Machine in Canada: The Pacification of the North*. Montreal: Black Rose Books, 1973.

Department of Indian Affairs, "Correspondence relating to tuberculous among the Indians in the various agencies across Canada 1908–1910." File 140, 754-1, DIA Archives.

Department of Indian Affairs, Superintendent D.C. Scott to Indian Agent General Major D. McKay, RG 1-Series, 12 April 1910, DIA Archives.

Deskaheh. "The Last Speech of Deskaheh." 1917. *Indymedia*. Rochester, NY, http://rochester.indymedia.org/node/878.

Dumont, Albert. *Broad Winged Hawk: A Book of Poetry and Short Stories*. Ottawa: Turtle Moons Press, 2007.

Dumont, Albert. *Of Trees and Their Wisdom: Poetry and Short Stories*. Ottawa: Turtle Moons Press, 2009.

Elsey, Christine J., *The Poetics of Land and Identity Among British Columbia Indigenous Peoples*. Halifax, Winnipeg: Fernwood Publishing, 2013.

Fear-Segal, Jacqueline, and Rebecca Tillett (eds.). *Indigenous Bodies; Reviewing, Relocating, Reclaiming*. Albany: State University of New York, 2013.

"First Nations Authors Discuss Carolyn Bennett's Indigenous Book Club Month." By Connie Walker. *The Current*, CBC Radio. January 8, 2016.

Fontaine, Theodore. *Broken Circle: The Dark Legacy of Indian Residential Schools, a Memoir*. Victoria: Heritage House, 2010.

Freire, Paulo. *Pedagogy of the Oppressed*. New York: Continuum, 2000.

Frolick, Larry. *Crow Never Dies: Life on the Great Hunt*. Edmonton: University of Alberta Press, 2016.

Fry, Alan. *How a People Die: A Novel*. Toronto: Doubleday Canada, 1970.

Gaudin, S.D. *Forty-four Years with the Northern Crees*. Toronto: Mundy-Goodfellow, 1942.

Gayles, Jonathan. Review of *The Great White North?* in *International Journal of Multicultural Education* 10, no. 2 (2008): 1–3.

Geddes, Gary. *Drink the Bitter Root: A Writer's Search for Justice and Redemption in Africa*. Vancouver: Douglas & McIntyre, 2011.

Geddes, Gary. "When the Cure is Worse." *This*. October 26, 2015, https://this.org/2015/10/26/when-the-cure-is-worse/.

Geddes, Gary. *Skookum Wawa: Writings of the Canadian Northwest*. Toronto: Oxford University Press, 1975.

Goldie, Terry. *Fear and Temptation: The Image of the Indigene in Canadian, Australian and New Zealand Literatures*. Kingston: McGill-Queen's University Press, 1989.

Goldrick-Jones, Amanda, and Herbert Rosengarten (eds). *The Broadview Anthology of Poetry*. Peterborough: Broadview Press, 1993.

Goodfellow, Anne Marie. *Talking in Context: Language and Identity in Kwakwa̱ka̱'wakw Society*. Montreal: McGill-Queen's University Press, 2005.

Goodman, Amy. "Idle No More: Indigenous-Led Protests Sweep Canada for Native Sovereignty and Environmental Justice." *Democracynow.org*, December 26, 2012, https://www.democracynow.org/2012/12/26/idle_no_more_indigenous_led_protests.

Grand Council Treaty #3. "Submission to the Ipperwash Inquiry." *The Ipperwash Inquiry, The Honourable Sidney B. Linden, Commissioner*. May 31, 2007.

Grant, Agnes. *Finding My Talk: How Fourteen Native Women Reclaimed Their Lives After Residential School*. Calgary: Fifth House, 2004.

Grant, Peter. "An Interview with Colin Brown." *Pacific Rim Review of Books* 11, vol. 5.2 (2009), http://www.prrb.ca/articles/issue11-grant.htm.

Grygier, Pat Sandiford. *A Long Way from Home: The Tuberculosis Epidemic Among the Inuit*. Mcgill-Queen's/Associated Medical Services Studies in the History of Medicine, Health, and Society, No. 2. Kingston: McGill-Queen's University Press, 1994.

Haig-Brown, Celia. *Resistance and Renewal: Surviving the Indian Residential School.* Vancouver: Arsenal Press, 1998.

Hardin, Herschel. *A Nation Unaware: The Canadian Economic Culture.* Vancouver: J.J. Douglas, 1974.

Harkin, Michael. "Contested Bodies: Affliction and Power in Heiltsuk Culture and History." *American Ethnologist* 21, no. 3 (1994): 586–604.

Harpster, John W. *Crossroads: Descriptions of Western Pennsylvania 1720–1829.* Pittsburgh: University of Pittsburgh Press, 1986 (1938).

Harrison, Klisala. "'Singing My Spirit of Identity': Aboriginal Music for Well-being in a Canadian Inner City." *MUSIcultures* 36 (2009): 1–21.

Henderson, J., and P. Wakeham. "Colonial Reckoning, National Reconciliation? First Peoples and the Culture of Redress in Canada." *English Studies in Canada* 35, no. 1 (2009): 1–26.

Henry, Kevin. "Colonialism Is a Public Health Problem." *Ricochet.* May 3, 2016, https://ricochet.media/en/1140/colonialism-is-a-public-health-problem.

Hogue, Michael. *Metis and the Medicine Line: Creating A Border and Dividing a People.* Chapel Hill: The University of North Carolina Press, 2015. https://www.attorney-general.jus.gov.on.ca/inquiries/ipperwash/policy_part/projects/pdf/Chiefs_of_Ontario-Grand_Council_Treaty_3.pdf.

Hutchison, George, and Dick Wallace. *Grassy Narrows.* Toronto: Van Nostrand Reinhold, 1977.

Inglis, Jasmine. "Yuxweluptun, Nicolson and Assu: Land, Environment and Activist Art in British Columbia." MA thesis, Carleton University, 2016.

Jenness, Diamond. *The Indians of Canada.* 1932. Toronto: University of Toronto Press, 1977.

Johnson, Kevin. "Toughness on Crime Gives Way to Fairness, Cost Reality." *USA Today.* March 30, 2014.

Kelm, Mary-Ellen. *Colonizing Bodies: Aboriginal Health and Healing in British Columbia, 1900–50.* Vancouver: UBC Press, 1998.

Kinew, Wab. "Interview with Pam Palmater—Candidate for AFN National Chief." *NetNewsLedger.* Posted June 27, 2012, http://www.netnewsledger.com/2012/06/27/interview-pam-palmater-candidate-afn-nationa-chief/.

Kinew, Wab. *The Reason You Walk.* Toronto: Viking, 2015.

King, Thomas. *The Inconvenient Indian: A Curious Account of Native People in North America.* Minneapolis: University of Minnesota Press, 2012.

Krotz, Larry. "A Canadian Genocide?" *UCObserver.* March 2014, http://www.ucob-server.org/features/2014/03/canadian_genocide/.

Kulchyski, Peter K. *Like the Sound of a Drum: Aboriginal Cultural Politics in Denendeh and Nunavut.* Winnipeg: University of Manitoba Press, 2005.

Kuper Island, Return to the Healing Circle (film). Victoria: Gumboot Productions, 1997.

Kundera, Milan. *The Book of Laughter and Forgetting: A Novel.* New York: Knopf, 1980.

Laird, David, J.H. Ross, and J.A.J. McKenna. Report of Indian Treaty Commissioners for Treaty No. 8. Winnipeg, MA, 22 September 1899, https://www.aadnc-aandc.gc.ca/eng/1100100028813/1100100028853.

Law, Stephanie. "State of Care Documentary: Canada's Segregated Health Care." *The Current*, CBC Radio, January 30, 2013, http://www.cbc.ca/radio/thecurrent/jan-30-2013-1.2910405/state-of-care-documentary-canada-s-segregated-health-care-1.2910408.

Lévi-Strauss, Claude. "A Writing Lesson," in *Tristes tropiques*. Trans. by John Russell. New York: Criterion, 1961, 290–93.

Ljunggren, David. "Every G20 Nation Wants to Be Canada, Insists PM." *Reuters*. September 25, 2009, http://www.reuters.com/article/columns-us-g20-canada-advantages-idUSTRE58P05Z20090926.

Loyie, Larry, Wayne K. Spear, and Constance Brissenden. *Residential Schools: With the Words and Images of Survivors*. Brantford: Indigenous Education Press, 2014.

Lutz, Hartmut. *Contemporary Challenges: Conversations with Canadian Native Authors*. Saskatoon: Fifth House, 1991.

Lux, Maureen Katherine. *Medicine That Walks: Disease, Medicine, and Canadian Plains Native People, 1880–1940*. Toronto: University of Toronto Press, 2001.

Lux, Maureen Katherine. *Separate Beds: A History of Indian Hospitals in Canada, 1920s–1980s*. Toronto: University of Toronto Press, 2016.

Maher, Stephen. "Not Genocide? Ask the Beothuks," *The National Post*, June 11, 2005, http://news.nationalpost.com/full-comment/stephen-maher-not-genocide-ask-the-beothuk.

Malacrida, Claudia. *A Special Hell: Institutional Life in Alberta's Eugenic Years*. Toronto: University of Toronto Press, 2015.

Mallinder, Lorraine. "Grim History of Canada's Racially Segregated Hospitals." *The Irish Times*. May 28, 2013, http://www.irishtimes.com/life-and-style/grim-history-of-canada-s-racially-segregated-hospitals-1.1407751?page=1.

Maracle, Lee. *Sojourners and Sundogs: First Nations Fiction*. Vancouver: Press Gang Publishers, 1999.

Marks, John. *The Search for the "Manchurian Candidate."* New York: Times Books, 1979.

Mast, Meghan, and Sam Fenn. "The Sisters of St. Ann." *The Terry Project on CiTR* (podcast). #37, April 24, 2014, http://www.terry.ubc.ca/2014/04/24/terry-project-37-the-sisters-of-saint-ann/.

Maté, Gabor. "How Do We Heal Trauma Suffered by Native Communities?" *Native Sun News Today*. April 20, 2016.

Maté, Gabor. "Psychedelics and Unlocking the Unconscious, from Cancer to Addiction." *Alternet*. May 30, 2013, http://www.alternet.org/drugs/gabor-mate-ayahuasca-maps-conference-2013.

Maud, Velvet. "Understanding Narratives of Illness and Contagion as a Strategy to Prevent Tuberculosis Among Métis in Southern Manitoba," MA thesis, University of Saskatchewan, 2012, http://hdl.handle.net/10388/ETD-2012-10-756.

McMahon, Ryan. "Red Man Laughing: The Wab Kinew Interview." *The Red Man Laughing Podcast*. Season 5, October 30, 2015, https://www.redmanlaughing.com/listen/2015/10/red-man-laughing-the-wab-kinew-interview.

McMillan, Alan D., and Eldon Yellowhorn. *First Peoples in Canada*. Vancouver: Douglas & McIntyre, 2004.

Meijer Drees, Laurie. *Healing Histories: Stories from Canada's Indian Hospitals*. Edmonton: University of Alberta Press, 2013.

Miller, J.R. *Shingwauk's Vision: A History of Native Residential Schools*. Toronto: University of Toronto Press, 1996.

Milloy, John S. *A National Crime: The Canadian Government and the Residential School System 1879 to 1986*. Winnipeg: University of Manitoba Press, 1999.

Mitchell, Catherine. "Perspective: 57 Years of Silence." *Winnipeg Free Press*. December 4, 2009, http://www.winnipegfreepress.com/local/57-years-of-silence-42868487.html.

Miyagawa, Mitch. *A Sorry State* (documentary film). CMF/FMC, 2014. https://www. knowledge.ca/program/sorry-state.

Møller, Helle. "Tuberculosis and Colonialism: Current Tales about Tuberculosis and Colonialism in Nunavut." *Journal of Aboriginal Health* 6, no. 1 (2010): 38–48.

Monture-Angus, Patricia. *Thunder in My Soul: A Mohawk Women Speaks.* Black Point, NS: Fernwood Publishing, 1995.

Morris, Alexander. *The Treaties of Canada with the Indians of Manitoba and the North- west Territories: Including the Negotiations on Which They Were Based, and Other Information Relating Thereto.* Chicago, New York, and San Fransisco: Belford, Clark & Company, 1880.

Mosby, Ian. "Administering Colonial Science: Nutrition Research and Human Biomedical Experimentation in Aboriginal Communities and Residential Schools, 1942–1952." *Social History* 46, no. 1 (2013): 145–172.

Mosby Ian. "Of History and Headlines: Reflections of an Accidental Public Historian." *Ian Mosby.ca* (blog). April 29, 2014, http://www.ianmosby.ca/of-history-and-headlines-reflections-of-an-accidental-public-historian/.

Moses, Daniel David, and Terry Goldie. *An Anthology of Canadian Native Literature in English.* Toronto: Oxford University Press, 2005.

"Nanaimo Indian Hospital." Interview with Joan Morris. *Nanaimo Daily News.* Uploaded December 15, 2011, to NanaimoDailyNews channel, https://youtu.be/ ZUOuUo79zU8.

Nanetti, Andrea, and Siew Ann Cheong. "The World as Seen from Venice (1205– 1533) as a Case Study of Scalable Web-Based Automatic Narratives for Interactive Global Histories." *The Asian Review of World Histories* 4, no. 1 (January 2016): 3–34.

Official Debates of the House of Commons of the Dominion of Canada, 4th Session, 4th Parliament, Vol. 12 (1882). Ottawa: Maclean, Roger & Co., 1882.

Painted Land: In Search of the Group of Seven (documentary film). White Pine Pictures, 2016.

Palmater, Pamela. "Canada Was Killing Indians, Not Culture." *telesurtv.* June 8, 2015, http://www.telesurtv.net/english/opinion/Canada-Was-Killing-Indians-Not-Cultures-20150608-0018.html.

Palmater, Pamela. "Canadian and Church Officials Must Be Held Accountable for Genocide." *telesurtv.* June 17, 2015, http://www.telesurtv.net/english/opinion/ Canadian-and-Church-Officials-Must-be-Accountable-for-Genocide-20150617-0033.html.

Palmater, Pamela. *Indigenous Nationhood: Empowering Grassroots Citizens.* Black Point, NS: Fernwood Publishing, 2015.

Palmer Gordon, Katherine. *We Are Born with the Songs Inside Us: Lives and Stories of First Nations People in British Columbia.* Madeira Park: Harbour, 2013.

Porter, Jody. "Dying for An Education: Little Charlie." *CBC Radio* (Thunder Bay). CBC, September 3, 2015: http://www.cbc.ca/news/dying-for-an-education-little-charlie-1.1732575.

Porter, Jody. "Ear Experiments Done on Kids at Kenora Residential School." *CBC News.* CBC, August 8, 2013, http://www.cbc.ca/news/canada/thunder-bay/ear-experiments-done-on-kids-at-kenora-residential-school-1.1343992.

Porter, Jody. 'Indian Hospital' Survivors Want Hospital Added to the Residential School Settlement Agreement." *CBC Radio (Thunder Bay).* December 29, 2014.

Purvis, Michael. "Getting the Whole Story of Shingwauk School." *The Sault Star.* June 28, 2015, http://www.saultstar.com/2009/08/26/getting-the-whole-story-of-shingwauk-school.

Quinn, Mark. "Residential School Students Still Want Apology, Compensation." *CBC News.* September 28, 2015, http://www.cbc.ca/news/canada/newfoundland-labrador/residential-school-students-still-want-apology-compensation-1.3245841.

Ralston Saul, John. *The Comeback.* Toronto: Viking, 2014.

Ray, Arthur J. *I Have Lived Here Since the World Began: An Illustrated History of Canada's Native People.* Montreal: McGill-Queen's University Press, 2011.

Regan, Paulette. *Unsettling the Settler Within: Indian Residential Schools, Truth Telling, and Reconciliation in Canada.* Vancouver: UBC Press, 2010.

Reilly, John. *Bad Judgment: The Myth of First Nations Equality and Judicial Independence in Canada.* Victoria: Rocky Mountain Books, 2014.

Reilly, John. *Bad Medicine: A Judge's Struggle for Justice in a First Nations Community.* Victoria: Rocky Mountain Books, 2010.

Ricou, Laurie. *Salal: Listening for the Northwest Understory.* Edmonton: NeWest Press, 2007.

Roberts, Charles G.D. *In Divers Tones.* 1886. Reprint, n.p.: Read Books, 2016.

Robertson, Heather. *Reservations Are for Indians.* Toronto: J. Lewis & Samuel, 1970.

Ross, Malcolm Mackenzie (ed.). *Poets of the Confederation: Duncan Campbell Scott, Archibald Lampman, Bliss Carman, Charles G.D. Roberts.* Toronto: McClelland & Stewart, 1960.

Ross, Malcolm Mackenzie. *The Impossible Sum of Our Traditions: Reflections on Canadian Literature.* Vancouver: McClelland & Stewart, 1986.

Ross, Rupert. *Indigenous Healing: Exploring Traditional Paths.* Toronto: Penguin, 2014.

Savage, Candace. *A Geography of Blood: Unearthing Memory from a Prairie Landscape.* Vancouver: Greystone Books, 2012.

Sellars, Bev. *They Called Me Number One: Secrets and Survival at an Indian Residential School.* Vancouver: Talonbooks, 2013.

Sellers, Patricia. Human and Ecological Health in Asubpeeschoseewagong Netum Anishinabek (Grassy Narrows First Nation). Report prepared for the ANA-Ontario Mercury Working Group, 2014.

Selway, Shawn. *Nobody Here Will Harm You: Mass Evacuations from the Eastern Arctic, 1950–1965.* Hamilton: James St North Books, 2015.

Shkilnyk, Anastasia M. *A Poison Stronger Than Love: The Destruction of an Ojibwa Community.* New Haven: Yale University Press, 1985.

Simpson, Leanne, and Kiera L. Ladner (eds.). *This Is an Honour Song: Twenty Years Since the Blockades, an Anthology of Writing on the "Oka Crisis."* Winnipeg: Arbeiter Ring, 2010.

Sinclair, Niigaanwewidam James, and Warren Cariou(eds.). *Manitowapow: Aboriginal Writings from the Land of Water.* Winnipeg: HighWater Press, 2011.

Spear, Wayne K. "Indian Residential Schools: A Brief History of the Mush Hole." *Wayne K. Spear* (blog). January 22, 2010, http://waynekspear.com/2010/01/22/the-mush-hole/

Spitzer, Alan B. *Historical Truths and Lies about the Past: Reflections on Dewey, Dreyfus, de' Man, and Reagan.* Chapel Hill: University of North Carolina Press, 1996.

Stannard, David E. *American Holocaust: Columbus and the Conquest of the New World.* New York: Oxford University Press, 1993.

Statues of the Province of Alberta 1928 Passed in the 2nd Session of the 6th Legislative Assembly. Edmonton: King's Printer, 1928.

Stonefish, Brent. *Moving Beyond: Understanding the Impacts of Residential School*. Owen Sound, ON: Ningwakwe Learning Press, 2007.

Storie, Suzanne, and Jennifer Gould(eds.). "Bella Bella Stories: Told by the People of Bella Bella." Unpublished manuscript, BC Indian Advisory Committee, Victoria, BC, 1973.

Stote, Karen. *An Act of Genocide: Colonialism and the Sterilization of Aboriginal Women*. Black Point, NS: Fernwood Publishing, 2015.

Stote, Karen. "The Coercive Sterilization of Aboriginal Women in Canada." *American Indian and Culture Research Journal* 36, no. 3 (2012): 117–150, doi:http://dx.doi.org/10.17953/aicr.36.3.7280728r6479j650.

Swanky, Tom. *The True Story of Canada's "War" of Extermination on the Pacific, Plus The Tsilhqot'in and Other First Nations Resistance*. Burnaby: Dragon Heart Enterprises, 2012.

Sylvester, Kevin. "The Story of a Separate and Unequal Canadian Health Care System." Interview with Maureen Lux. *The Sunday Edition*, CBC, August 5, 2016, http://www.cbc.ca/radio/thesundayedition/revolver-at-50-canada-s-history-of-segregated-healthcare-frog-march-firings-penny-lang-1.3707673/the-story-of-a-separate-and-unequal-canadian-health-care-system-1.3707678.

The Invisible Nation (film). Directed by Richard Desjardin and Robert Monderie. National Film Board of Canada, 2012.

Thompson, Nancy. "Watson Lake Families Seek Answers from Yukon Hospital Corp." *CBC News* (North). November 26, 2013, http://www.cbc.ca/news/canada/north/watson-lake-families-seek-answers-from-yukon-hospital-corp-1.2440058.

Timpson, Annis May (ed.). *First Nations, First Thoughts: The Impact of Indigenous Thought in Canada*. Vancouver: UBC Press, 2009.

Turner, Nancy J. *The Earth's Blanket*. New York: Douglas & McIntyre, 2008.

Turner, Nancy J., and Katherine L. Turner. "'Where Our Women Used to Get the Food': Cumulative Effects and Loss of Ethnobotanical Knowledge and Practice; Case Study from Coastal British Columbia." *Botany* 86, no. 2 (2008): 103–115, doi:10.1139/B07-020.

Turtle Island Native Network, http://www.turtleisland.org/resources/resources001.htm.

Tyman, James. *Inside Out: An Autobiography of a Native Canadian*. Saskatoon: Fifth House, 1989.

Wagamese, Richard. *Indian Horse*. Vancouver: Douglas & McIntyre, 2012.

Wagamese, Richard. *Medicine Walk*. Toronto: McClelland and Stewart, 2014.

Wagamese, Richard. "Witholding Stories Denies the Truths." *Eagle Feather News* 16, no. 8 (August 2013): 16.

Waldram, James B., D. Ann Herring, and T. Kue Young. *Aboriginal Health in Canada: Historical, Cultural, and Epidemiological Perspectives*. Toronto: University of Toronto Press, 2006.

Wilson, Milton (ed.). *Poetry of Mid-Century 1940–1960*. Toronto: McClelland and Stewart, 1964.

Wolfson, Carmelle. "How Grassy Narrows Lawsuit Could Change Aboriginal–Government Relations Across Canada." *This*. November 22, 2011, https://this.org/2011/11/22/grassy-narrows/.

Wu, David. "An Interview with Elder Fred John, Part 1." *Caring for Our Children* (news-letter), *BC Aboriginal Care Society* 13, no. 5 (Jan-Feb 2011), http://www.acc-society.bc.ca/files_new/documents/CFOCJan-Feb11Final.pdf.

Wu, David. "Traditional Drumming and Cultural Healing: An Interview with Fred John, Part 2." *Caring for Our Children* (newsletter), *BC Aboriginal Care Society* 13, no. 6 (March-April, 2011), http://www.acc-society.bc.ca/files_new/documents/CFOCMar-Apr11.pdf.

York, Geoffrey. *The Dispossessed: Life and Death in Native Canada*. Toronto: Lester & Orpen Dennys, 1989.

Index

In this index page numbers set in italics indicate a photograph.

Also by Gary Geddes

POETRY

Poems (1971)
Rivers Inlet (1972)
Snakeroot (1973)
Letter of the Master of Horse (1973)
War & Other Measures (1976)
The Acid Test (1980)
The Terracotta Army (1984; 2007; 2010)
Changes of State (1986)
Hong Kong (1987)
No Easy Exit (1989)
Light of Burning Towers (1990)
Girl by the Water (1994)
The Perfect Cold Warrior (1995)
Active Trading: Selected Poems 1970–1995 (1996)
Flying Blind (1998)
Skaldance (2004)
Falsework (2007)
Swimming Ginger (2010)
What Does a House Want? (2014)
The Resumption of Play (2016)

FICTION

The Unsettling of the West (1986)

NON-FICTION

Letters from Managua: Meditations on Politics & Art (1990)
Sailing Home: A Journey through Time, Place & Memory (2001)
Kingdom of Ten Thousand Things: An Impossible Journey from Kabul to Chiapas (2005)
Drink the Bitter Root: A Search for Justice and Healing in Africa (2010; USA, 2011)

DRAMA

Les Maudits Anglais (1984)

TRANSLATIONS

I Didn't Notice the Mountain Growing Dark (1986), poems of Li Bai and Du Fu, translated with the assistance of George Liang

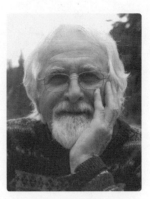

About the Author

Gary Geddes is a bestselling author and the winner of more than a dozen national and international literary awards. He has written and edited more than forty-five books of poetry, fiction, drama, non-fiction, criticism, translation, and anthologies. His prestigious awards include the Commonwealth Poetry Prize (Americas Region), the Writers Choice Award, the National Magazine Gold Award, the Lieutenant-Governor's Award for Literary Excellence, and the Gabriela Mistral Prize, awarded simultaneously to Nobel laureates Octavio Paz and Vaclav Havel, as well as to Ernesto Cardenal, Rafael Alberti, and Mario Benedetti. His other non-fiction works include the bestselling *Sailing Home, Kingdom of Ten Thousand Things*, and *Drink the Bitter Root*, which was shortlisted for the Hubert Evans Non-fiction Prize. He lives on Thetis Island, British Columbia.